BTLS:
BASIC PREHOSPITAL TRAUMA CARE

BTLS:
BASIC PREHOSPITAL TRAUMA CARE

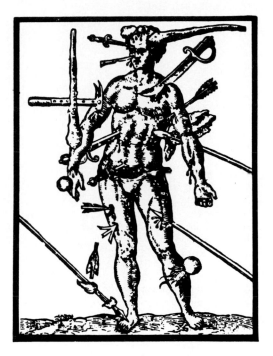

John Emory Campbell, M.D.

Alabama Chapter, American College
of Emergency Physicians

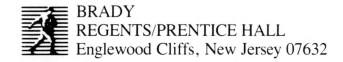

BRADY
REGENTS/PRENTICE HALL
Englewood Cliffs, New Jersey 07632

Library of Congress Cataloging-in-Publication Data

Campbell, John E., 1943-
   BTLS : basic prehospital trauma care.

  "A Brady book."
  Includes index.
  1. Emergency medicine. 2. Wounds and injuries.
I. Title. [DNLM: 1. Allied Health Personnel.
2. Emergency Medical Services. 3. Wounds and Injuries.
WX 215 C188ba]
RC86.7.C342 1988   617´.1026   88-4183
ISBN 0-89303-122-4 (pbk.)

Editorial/production supervision and
  interior design: Eileen M. O'Sullivan
Manufacturing buyer: Bob Anderson
Page layout: Karen Salzbach

© 1988 by Prentice-Hall, Inc.
A Simon & Schuster Company
Englewood Cliffs, New Jersey 07632

Printed in the United States of America

10 9 8

ISBN   0-89303-122-4

PRENTICE-HALL INTERNATIONAL (UK) LIMITED, *London*
PRENTICE-HALL OF AUSTRALIA PTY. LIMITED, *Sydney*
PRENTICE-HALL CANADA INC., *Toronto*
PRENTICE-HALL HISPANOAMERICANA, S.A., *Mexico*
PRENTICE-HALL OF INDIA PRIVATE LIMITED, *New Delhi*
PRENTICE-HALL OF JAPAN, INC., *Tokyo*
SIMON & SCHUSTER ASIA PTE. LTD., *Singapore*
EDITORA PRENTICE-HALL DO BRASIL, LTDA., *Rio de Janeiro*

To Jackie, Pat, Ray, Casey, Jason, and the whole BTLS FAMILY. . . .
Thanks!
I could not have done it without you.

This book is dedicated to Captain Jim McClellan and the Clay County Rescue Squad. Many years ago when I was a young doctor impressed with my own importance, I had the honor of working with them. I taught them some basic EMT skills and they taught me about humility and unselfish devotion to humankind. Over the years they have not only provided Clay County, Alabama with the finest in prehospital care, but have also provided me a standard of character and dedication with which to measure my own life.

CONTENTS

FOREWORD   *xi*

INTRODUCTION   *xiii*

CHAPTERS

1   TRAUMA CARE IN PERSPECTIVE   *1*

2   MECHANISMS OF MOTION INJURY   *4*

3   INITIAL EVALUATION OF THE TRAUMA VICTIM   *22*

4   MANAGING THE AIRWAY   *43*

5   CHEST TRAUMA   *59*

6   SHOCK   *75*

7   SPINAL CORD TRAUMA   *85*

8   HEAD TRAUMA   *99*

9   ABDOMINAL TRAUMA   *114*

10   EXTREMITY TRAUMA   *120*

11 BURNS   140

12 TRAUMA IN PREGNANCY   153

13 PEDIATRIC TRAUMA   161

14 CRITICAL TRAUMA SITUATIONS "LOAD AND GO"   169

SKILL STATIONS

1 UPPER AIRWAY MANAGEMENT   173

2 SPINAL IMMOBILIZATION—SHORT BACKBOARD   181

3 EMERGENCY RAPID EXTRICATION   189

4 TRACTION SPLINTS   194

5 APPLICATION OF THE ANTISHOCK GARMENT   201

6 HELMET REMOVAL   207

7 LONG BACKBOARD   211

8 PRIMARY SURVEY   224

9 SECONDARY SURVEY   236

10 RAPID PATIENT ASSESSMENT   246

GLOSSARY   254

INDEX   259

FOREWORD

By
Ray Fowler, M.D., FACEP

At any moment something may happen that could take away a life, whether it be a high-speed head-on collision with a tree or the sudden onset of cardiac arrest. The development of closed chest massage in 1959 and the improved response of emergency medical teams in World War II, the Korean War, and the Vietnam War brought people and governments into an awareness that sudden life-threatening events could perhaps be survived. In the 1960s and 1970s systems were developed around the world to deliver emergency care to citizens wherever they might be in distress.

The growth of emergency medicine as a specialty in the last decade has provided the final link between injury and the provision of first aid. Everyone involved in the provision of emergency medicine has gradually come to be scrutinized closely as to the quality of the care that they provide.

In the late 1970s and early 1980s it became apparent to John Campbell that there was a significant gap between the daily responsibilities of EMS personnel and the training provided to fulfill these duties. John saw the positive results of the American Heart Association's program on cardiac emergencies and the American College of Surgeons' program on trauma assessment and management for physicians. The two-day lecture and skill station format impressed him as a useful tool for bringing pertinent knowledge and techniques to a target audience. With a will that comes only from sincere commitment, John, his wife Jackie, and the training coordinator for the local EMS region, Pat Gandy, conceived, designed, and implemented a prototype program and set it in motion in Opelika, Alabama. What followed is history.

Within four years over half of the United States as well as Canada and Puerto Rico had established Basic Trauma Life Support organizations to provide this critical knowledge to field and emergency department personnel. The Instructor and Provider texts were being published by Brady. A national consensus organization was established for future advancement of the course materials as well as for quality assurance of the educational efforts.

The great success of Basic Trauma Life Support refocused John's thinking on the educational gap that started him on the BTLS path. He saw that BTLS was in many ways "advanced trauma care" in the field, including such procedures as endotracheal intubation, needle decompression of the chest, needle cricothyrotomy, and intravenous infusions. Such procedures made BTLS go beyond the training of the most common prehospital provider.

So John Campbell, together with his wife, went back to work for a year with a word processor and produced *BTLS: Basic Prehospital Care*. This authoritative text is for the EMT-A the "basic," the most widespread provider of emergency medicine in the field.

This course gleans from BTLS all of the fundamental principles of patient evaluation and management, eliminating advanced concepts and procedures that go beyond the training of the EMT-A. Its purpose is for two days to focus the basic EMT's concentration on what the acutely injured patient looks like, what the signs and symptoms are, what conclusions may be drawn from these symptoms and findings, and how these acute conditions should be managed.

Properly approached, this course will be the greatest professional challenge that basic EMTs will have in their training. This is as it should be. The major trauma patient has the greatest risk of dying, is the hardest patient to manage, and has the greatest chance of being saved. This text and program is for those basic EMTs who want to practice the best possible trauma care.

INTRODUCTION

The Basic Trauma Life Support Course for Paramedics was first taught in August 1982. In the intervening five years it has become the standard pre-hospital trauma training course for advanced EMTs and paramedics. *BTLS: Basic Prehospital Care* is designed to offer the same hands-on trauma training to the EMT-A. The experience of teaching 10,000 students has been incorporated into this material. The greatest difficulty encountered by most students has been patient assessment, thus the skills section of this course has been redesigned to add further emphasis on assessment skills. The other skill stations are presented using accepted methods and techniques in common use. It is recognized that there are other equally acceptable techniques to perform some of these skills and it is reasonable to modify these techniques to conform to the standard procedures in your area. Although this course has been designed for a 16-hour or two-day format, it can be taught effectively in small blocks over a longer period. Slides and an Instructor's Guide for use with this book are available to any educational organization. If you require assistance in arranging courses in your area, the national BTLS organization will be happy to help. Please write or call:

Basic Trauma Life Support　　　　　　　　　　　　　　(205) 567-2000
P.O. Box 210727
Montgomery, Alabama 36121-0727

BTLS:
BASIC PREHOSPITAL TRAUMA CARE

PART I

Chapter 1

TRAUMA CARE IN PERSPECTIVE

The leading causes of death in the United States are heart disease, cancer, and stroke. Millions of dollars are spent each year in search of methods to prevent or cure these most dreaded diseases. Overlooked in the effort to reduce mortality from disease is the fact that the major health problem facing young Americans is trauma. Among children and young adults, death and disability are much more commonly due to physical injury (trauma) than to any medical illness. Trauma is the leading cause of death of all Americans from age 1 through age 44. In contrast to cancer and cardiovascular diseases, trauma is both readily preventable and treatable. Sadly, very little money or resources have been committed to the goals of preventing or curing injuries. Only in the last two decades have we begun seriously to study methods of trauma care.

During the Vietnam War the military made great strides in the treatment of trauma. They proved that rapid trauma care saves lives. Using specially trained field medics (the forerunners of paramedics), rapid pickup and transport by helicopter, and special surgical hospitals, they were able to decrease dramatically the mortality rate for battlefield trauma, to the lowest in history (2 percent). In the civilian sector, Dr. R. Adams Cowley began the now famous Shock-Trauma Unit in Baltimore, Maryland. One of his most important discoveries was that survival from major trauma is directly related to the speed of definitive (surgical) treatment. He says: "You think people die from accidents or from heart attacks, but they really don't, not directly. Those things produce shock, which is sluggish or nonexistent circulation, and that's what kills you. Maybe you'll die in 10 minutes or maybe you'll die next week, but you're dead. So if you're in shock we have to work fast. You've got, at most, 60 minutes. If I can get to you, stop your bleeding, and restore your blood pressure within an hour of your accident . . . then I can probably save you. I call this the golden hour.'' Dr. Cowley found that if the seriously injured victim was in the operating room within an hour of his injury the death rate was about 15 percent. This rate doubled for every hour lost in getting to surgery. Operating within this time frame requires teamwork not only with responders and EMTs in the prehospital phase of emergency care but also with personnel in the emergency department, surgery department, and often even between hospitals.

The National EMS (Emergency Medical Services) Systems Act was passed in 1973. This set up 300 EMS regions across the country and provided grants to develop them. This seed money has resulted in most states now having well-established regional EMS systems. The goals of the regional EMS agencies are the planning and development of organized emergency care. In the prehospital phase, this often involves organizing, training, and equipping rescue units. Unfortunately, lack of funds have often prevented many rural systems from being well trained or well equipped. Enthusiasm and dedication are usually the only resources that are abundant. These rural areas are frequently provided rescue and ambulance services by volunteer organizations whose members have little time or money to invest in advanced life support training or equipment. The dedicated basic EMT (Emergency Medical Technician) is the backbone of these systems as well as many private and municipal ambulance services.

The majority of all prehospital trauma care in this country is still provided by the basic EMT. In order to decrease the devastating effects of trauma, practical trauma training must be made available to basic EMTs so that they can maximize the chances of the victims they serve. Although basic EMTs may feel that their training and capabilities are limited, they are indeed capable of providing lifesaving prehospital trauma care. Actually, advanced life support procedures are not as important as accurate assessment, rapid packaging, and efficient transport. Well-trained basic EMTs are not at a great disadvantage in providing prehospital trauma care.

Basic EMTs who serve with more advanced EMTs are an important part of the trauma team. Advanced procedures other than endotracheal intubation and intravenous fluids are rarely used on the trauma victim. Basic skills are used much more frequently, so basic EMTs should take pride in learning and performing them well. The EMT who is superbly trained in basic procedures is more effective in saving lives than a paramedic who is indecisive about when or how to perform advanced lifesaving techniques. Trauma care is a team sport like football—and just as in football, the team that best performs the basics usually wins.

Chapter 2

MECHANISMS OF MOTION INJURY

Many potentially fatal injuries are not apparent immediately. If you suspect and are prepared for the treatment of such injuries, you will often save that person's life. The ability to predict possible injuries by trauma scene assessment is an important skill and one that requires study, experience, and constant awareness to master. Although there are many other mechanisms of injury (electrocution, airway obstruction, toxic inhalation, etc.), motion injuries are most common. Motion injuries are due to transfer of energy from movement of the patient or objects that act on the patient. There are certain laws of physics with which you must become familiar in order to understand the transfer of energy.

Newton's first law of motion: A body at rest remains at rest unless acted upon by an outside force.

Newton's second law of motion: A body in motion remains in motion in a straight line unless acted upon by an outside force.

Injuries caused by the starting or stopping of motion are from the transfer of energy. Energy must be applied to an object at rest in order to make it move, and energy must be applied to an object in motion to make it stop.

The amount of energy applied, how quickly it is applied, and to what part of the body that energy is applied determines how much and how serious the injury will be.

EXAMPLE: An automobile (and its occupants) traveling at 60 miles per hour has a tremendous amount of mechanical energy. If this car hits a tree and is brought to an immediate stop, all of that energy must be absorbed by the tree, the auto, and the occupants. Serious injuries are likely to occur to the occupants because of this energy transfer. The same amount of energy is needed to stop the car by applying the brakes. No injuries occur as a result of slow deceleration by use of the brakes because the energy is converted to thermal energy by the friction of the brakes and this energy change occurs over a longer period. The transfer is hardly noticed by the occupants unless the brakes are applied too rapidly, in which case the auto will slow rapidly and the occupants will continue forward until they hit the steering wheel or dashboard.

The amount of energy produced by a body is equal to one-half the mass (weight) multiplied times the square of the velocity (speed).

Energy $= \frac{1}{2}$ Mass $\times$ Velocity^2

It is apparent that *speed* is more important than *weight* in the production of energy.

EXAMPLE: An M-16 rifle bullet weighing only 55 grains but traveling at 3200 ft per second causes *many* times the tissue damage as a .45-caliber pistol bullet weighing 230 grains but traveling only 810 ft per second. The rifle bullet, although only one-fifth the weight, produces *four times* the energy (1280 ft/lb versus 335 ft/lb) because of its speed.

All of this begins to sound very complicated, but once you grasp the basic principles you can readily apply them to the trauma scene. Questions you should try to answer at every trauma scene are:

1.   What happened?
2.   What sort of force (energy) was applied?
3.   To what part of the body and in what direction was the force applied?
4.   How much force was involved (speed, mass, weight)?

Organs inside the body obey Newton's laws also.

EXAMPLE: A person traveling at 30 miles per hour runs his car into a brick wall. The car stops immediately but the victim's body continues moving at 30 mph until his chest hits the steering wheel and his head hits the windshield. The brain tissue continues forward at 30 mph until it hits the inner surface of the skull. The heart and other internal organs continue forward at 30 mph until they impact some stationary object or until they are stopped by their ligamentous attachments.

Thus every deceleration (sudden stop) accident is a series of collisions, each capable of causing its own type of injury. When you survey the trauma scene you must reconstruct in your mind how the accident occurred in order to con-

Figure 2-1.

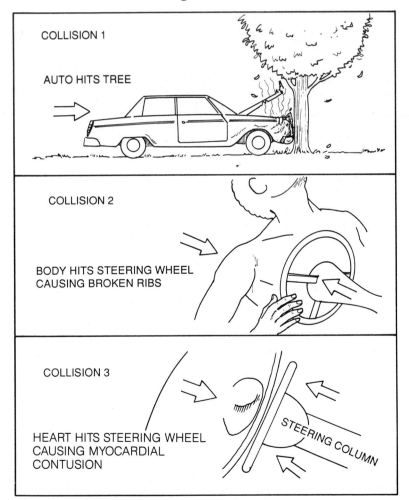

COLLISION 1

AUTO HITS TREE

COLLISION 2

BODY HITS STEERING WHEEL
CAUSING BROKEN RIBS

COLLISION 3

HEART HITS STEERING WHEEL
CAUSING MYOCARDIAL
CONTUSION

STEERING COLUMN

sider the forces involved and how they may have applied to the body of the victim. As you examine the victim you must look for the evidence of injury to the outside of the body and keep in mind the overall forces involved. Be suspicious for likely injuries inside the body. When you become good at this you will always be prepared for the early treatment of those injuries that may not have been apparent on first examination.

Application of Basic Principles to Specific Situations

I. **Large motor vehicle accidents**
Speed is the most important predictor of severity of injury. Other important factors are the direction from which the forces were applied and whether the occupants were restrained in their seats. Speed and this force (energy) may be estimated by looking at the damage to the vehicle itself. Severely damaged vehicles are more likely to have seriously injured occupants. This information should be relayed to the doctor in the emergency department. A description of the scene becomes more important when the car shows evidence of high impact forces (such as demolished car) but the occupant does not initially appear to have any serious injuries. This patient will need observation and frequent repeat surveys for possible hidden internal injuries.

A. *Frontal deceleration collisions:* When an automobile strikes a solid object and comes to an abrupt stop, the occupants inside will continue forward until they impact on some part of the auto. They may even be ejected and impact on some object outside the auto. Injuries sustained will depend on where the occupants are sitting and what they strike.

1. *Driver:* An unrestrained driver sitting high with his weight forward may be thrown upward, striking his head on the roof or windshield. His chest or abdomen will impact on the steering wheel and his legs may catch under the steering wheel as his body rises. Injuries to the head, neck, chest, abdomen, and femurs are likely in this situation. The driver who continues through the windshield and is ejected may sustain injuries to any part of the body since no one can predict exactly what may be hit during and after leaving the auto. A victim ejected from a car is 25 times as likely to be killed. This is not appreciated by most drivers, who persist in the foolish notion that being restrained by a seat belt makes them more likely to be trapped and killed in an auto accident.

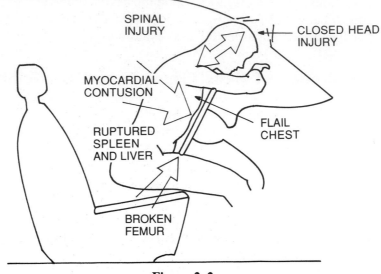

SPINAL
INJURY

CLOSED HEAD
INJURY

MYOCARDIAL
CONTUSION

FLAIL
CHEST

RUPTURED
SPLEEN
AND LIVER

BROKEN
FEMUR

Figure 2–2.

If the driver is sitting in a more extended position (common seating in low-slung sports-type autos), the body will more likely slide down under the steering wheel with the initial impact being through the feet and up the legs into the pelvis. The upper body will then swing forward, hitting the steering wheel. This victim will likely have fractures of the legs or pelvis as well as abdominal, chest, neck, and head injuries. Dislocation of the knee or hip is very common in this situation.

2. *Front-seat passenger:* The direction of forces is again either "up and over" or "down and under." The difference is that the steering wheel is not present. The body impacts the roof, windshield, dashboard, or floorboard. Injuries from head to foot can still occur.

3. *Rear-seat passengers:* These victims are in a little better position in that they impact the front seats and the front-seat passengers. Seats and passengers are somewhat less solid than are the dashboard and steering wheel. This may allow the energy to be dispersed over a longer time and distance, thus decreasing the severity of injuries. Do not let this keep you

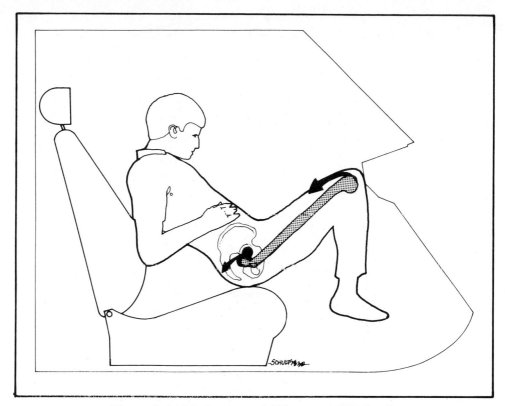

Figure 2–3. Mechanism of "Down and Under."

from suspecting the same types of injuries as may be found among front-seat passengers. When there are back-seat passengers, you must suspect more severe injuries among the front-seat passengers. Passengers in the front may have compression injuries from having been pinned between the steering wheel or dashboard and the backseat passengers. This is an example of three different mechanisms causing injuries. First the victim's body hits the inside of the auto, then the victim's internal organs impact, then the victim's body is compressed between another victim and the dashboard or steering wheel.

4. *Restrained occupants:* Restrained occupants are much more likely to survive because they are prevented from much of the impact inside the auto and they are prevented from being ejected from the auto. These occupants may sustain certain injuries. The lap belt is intended to go across the pelvis

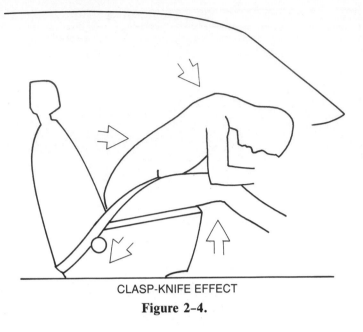

CLASP-KNIFE EFFECT

Figure 2-4.

(iliac crests), not the abdomen. If the belt is in place and the victim is subjected to a frontal deceleration accident, his body tends to fold together like a "clasp knife." The head may be thrown forward into the steering wheel or dashboard, so facial, head or neck injuries are common. Abdominal injuries occur if the lap belt is positioned improperly. Compression forces when the body is suddenly folded about the waist may injure the abdomen or the lumbar spine. The three-point restraint or cross chest–lap belt secures the body much better than the lap belt alone. The chest and pelvis are restrained, so life-threatening injuries are much less common. The head is not restrained, and therefore the neck is still subjected to stresses that may cause fractures, dislocations, or spinal cord injuries. Clavicular fractures (where the chest strap crosses) are common. Internal organ damage may still occur due to organ movement inside the body.

Air bags are designed to inflate from the center of the steering wheel and the dashboard to protect the front-seat occupants in case of a frontal deceleration accident. If these function properly, they cushion the head and chest at the instant

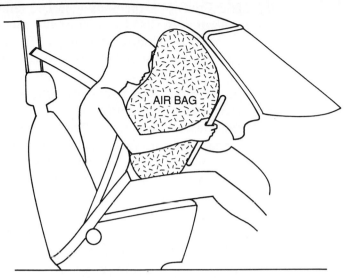

AIR BAG AND 3-POINT RESTRAINT

Figure 2–5.

of impact. This is very effective in decreasing injury to the face, neck, and chest. You should still immobilize the neck until it is adequately examined. Air bags deflate immediately so they protect against only one impact. A driver whose car hits more than one object is unprotected after the initial collision. They also do not prevent "down and under" movement, so drivers who are extended (tall drivers and drivers of small low-slung autos) may still impact with their legs and suffer leg, pelvis, or abdominal injuries. It is important for occupants to wear chest and lap belts even when the car is equipped with air bags.

B. *Lateral impact collisions:* When an auto is struck from the side, the effect is the same as a deceleration injury. In this case, the side of the victim's body is the impact area. Speed is still the major predictor of severity of injury, but the mass of the colliding object as well as the strength of construction of the vehicle in which the victim is riding also must be considered. A person riding in a heavy sedan struck in the side by a motorcycle would probably have fewer injuries than someone riding in a small economy car hit in the side by a truck.

When the collision occurs, the impact areas are usually the head, chest, pelvis, and often the arm and leg on the affected side. For all practical purposes the body is jerked laterally, so the head is first accelerated toward the side of the car, often impacting on the door pillar or window. The head is then jerked back to the opposite side. There may be head or neck injuries as a result of these movements. The lateral chest and arm impact against the inside of the door. This may cause rib, arm, or clavicular fractures, and internal injuries may arise from movement of the organs inside the chest and abdomen. The liver is frequently injured on victims struck on the right side, and the spleen is injured when the forces come from the left side. The impact forces tend to be focused at the level of the pelvis since this is the level at which an automobile bumper usually strikes the side of another auto. Fractures of the pelvis and/or upper leg frequently occur in significant lateral impact collisions. Seat restraints are not nearly so helpful in lateral impact accidents, but they do help hold the victim to his seat so that the car cannot shift out from under him when the collision occurs. Restraints help prevent the impact of the pelvis and upper leg against the inside of the door. Air bags are of no protection in this situation. If the lateral collision occurs at the front or the rear of the car, the forces become rotational with the car rotating around the point of impact. The forces exerted on the occupants are more of a combination of lateral and frontal deceleration. Seat restraints and air bags give good protection in preventing the occupants from being thrown about inside the car.

C. *Rear impact collisions:* In this situation, a stationary or slower-moving vehicle is hit from the rear, causing sudden acceleration forward. The body is usually well supported up to the level of the neck, so the forces acting on the body are not severe except above the shoulders. Properly positioned head rests support the head and neck and usually prevent serious neck or spinal injuries. Unfortunately, many head rests are not well designed and give no support or protection to any but the shortest people. The average person's neck and head is above the level of the head rests. When a sudden force is exerted from the rear, the body is accelerated forward and the head is accelerated backward, causing stretching and tearing of the supporting ligaments and muscles of the neck. Dislocation and/or fracture of the neck may occur. After the head accelerates backward, it is then snapped forward, causing further injury to the neck. This may be made worse if the car collides into the back of another car, causing the victim's en-

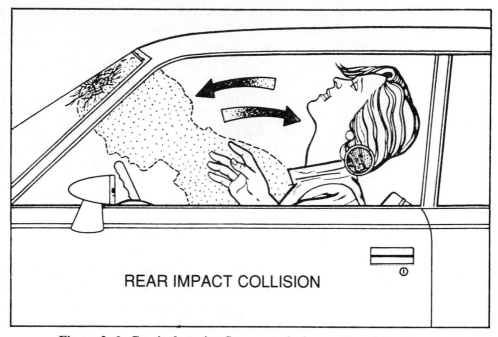

REAR IMPACT COLLISION

Figure 2–6. Cervical strain. Severe strain is usually evident from the history of the accident. Hyperextension or hyperflexion is often the mechanism of injury, which may involve either stretching or tearing of ligaments. Symptoms include neck immobility (caused by pain) and spasm of injured muscles.

tire body to be thrown forward, adding deceleration injuries to the rear impact injuries.

D. *Rollover accidents:* If the vehicle rolls over, there is no way to predict what forces will act on the occupants. You must always assume the possibility of both spinal and internal injuries. Occupants not wearing restraints are frequently ejected from the vehicle.

E. *Children in automobile accidents:* Unsecured children are at greater risk than adults in auto accidents. Most states now have laws requiring that small children be secured in special child restraint seats. Shamefully, many law enforcement officials disregard these laws and do not enforce them. Even minor accidents cause children to be thrown around inside the vehicle. The largest and heaviest part of the child, the head, usually impacts first, making head injuries common. In fact, trauma is the number one killer of children, and head injuries are the major cause of death from trauma in children. If a child is standing in the seat, his weight will be high and he will be thrown "up and over" into the windshield and perhaps ejected from the vehicle. If the child is sitting in an adult's lap, he will also be in danger because he may be crushed between the dashboard and the heavy body of the adult. Children allowed to play freely in the back of station wagons are at great risk from rear impact collisions. The children are accelerated through the rear window onto the roadway between the two vehicles. They may then be run over by the following vehicle. Mothers should be taught these facts during pregnancy. The time to begin to train a child in the use of infant restraint seats is soon after birth, on the ride home from the hospital (first ride-safe ride program).

F. *Auto–pedestrian accidents:* The pedestrian struck by a car almost always suffers severe internal injuries as well as fractures. This is true even if the vehicle is traveling at low speed. The mass of the auto is so large that high speed is not necessary to impart high-energy transfer. When high speed is involved the results are disastrous. There are two mechanisms of injury. The first is when the bumper of the auto strikes the body, and the second is when the body, accelerated by the transfer of forces strikes the ground or some other object. An adult usually has bilateral lower leg or knee fractures plus whatever secondary injuries occur when his body strikes the hood of the car and then later the ground. Children are shorter, so the bumper is more likely to hit them in the pelvis or torso. They usually land on their heads in the secondary impact. When answering a call to an auto–pedestrian accident, be prepared for broken bones, internal injuries, and head injuries.

G. *Tractor accidents:* Like three-wheeled ATVs, tractors are dangerous machines with a high center of gravity. They are easy to turn over and they frequently must be used on hillsides. One-third of all farm accident fatalities are due to tractor accidents. The majority of these fatal accidents are due to the machine tipping over and crushing the driver. Most overturns (85 percent) are to the side. These are less likely to pin the driver because he has a chance to jump or be thrown clear. Rear overturns, although less frequent, are more likely to crush the driver because he has almost no opportunity to jump free. The injuries are usually blunt trauma from being caught between the seat, wheels, and/or tractor body and the ground. The driver will frequently be trapped with his knees crushed against his chest. He will usually have major internal

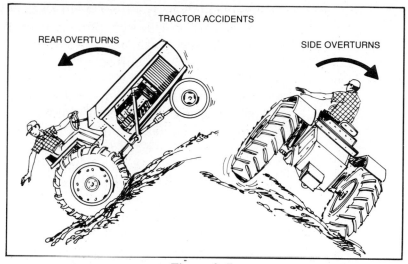

Figure 2–7.

injuries and may immediately go into shock from internal bleeding when you release the pressure on his abdomen. Further injuries are often chemical burns from gasoline, diesel fuel, hydraulic fluid, or even battery acid leaking onto the victim. There is a very real danger of fire from spilled gasoline. Rescue is often very difficult because tractors are heavy, with a tricky center of gravity. They are also usually overturned on soft ground. Occasionally, the tractor will shift as it is being lifted, crushing the driver a second time.

II. Small motor vehicle accidents

A. *Motorcycles:* Motorcycles are the most dangerous vehicles known. They provide no protection to their riders, are difficult to control, difficult to stop, and are often overlooked by other traffic. The rider can be thought of as a high-speed pedestrian. Where motorcycle riders are required to wear helmets, there is a decrease in the number of major head injuries (three times as many fatalities among those who do not wear helmets). Theoretically, among helmet-wearing riders, there should be more cervical spine injuries because the head is heavier with a helmet in place, thus increasing the magnitude of the forces acting on the neck.

   1. *Frontal deceleration collisions:* The weight of the rider is high, so the rider is thrown ''up and over'' the handlebars. Injuries to the genitalia and legs are common in the initial impact as the rider strikes the handlebars. The next collision is when

the victim's body strikes whatever is in his path (auto, tree, ground, etc.). This mechanism is much like being ejected from an auto; therefore, death rates from motorcycle accidents are very high. When confronted with an impending collision, experienced riders will turn the motorcycle to the side and lean away from the collision, causing the cycle to fall on its side and slide away from the rider into the collision. This will often prevent some major injuries, but the rider, unless wearing special protective clothes, will usually have severe abrasions (road rash) from head to feet.

2. *Lateral impact collisions:* Since there is no lateral protection, the rider is much the same as a pedestrian when struck from the side. If he survives, he will probably have major extremity and internal injuries. Amputations are quite common in this situation.

3. *Rear impact collisions:* Here again the rider is much like a pedestrian and will frequently have major extremity and internal injuries. Riders will often be run over by the vehicle that struck the motorcycle.

B. *Three-wheeled motorcycles (ATVs):* There is a major epidemic of injuries from the use of these very popular recreational all-terrain vehicles (ATVs). This has largely gone unnoticed in the major metropolitan areas because ATVs are generally used in rural areas. These vehicles are rarely ridden on public roads, so the mechanisms of injury are different than usually seen with two-wheeled motorcycles. ATVs have a high center of gravity and are difficult to steer because of the large fat front tire. Unless the rider shifts his weight correctly when turning, the vehicle frequently turns over. The balance required is different from that required on a bicycle or two-wheeled motorcycle. Experienced bicycle and two-wheeled motorcycle riders develop a natural tendency to put a foot down to support the bike when they stop. When a rider does this on an ATV, the rear tire will run over the foot, catching the leg and throwing the rider forward off the vehicle and onto his shoulder. Most injuries are to the extremities with fractures of the clavicle (falling on shoulder) being the most common. Many suffer fractures of the knee or lower leg from running into objects (difficult to steer). Head injuries are the major cause of fatal accidents (1 to 4 percent). ATV riders frequently do not wear helmets and these vehicles have a tendency to flip and fall on their riders. Because three-wheeled ATVs look like tricycles, the public has the mistaken impression that they are safe and easy to ride. It is sad but common to find children too young to ride a bicycle safely, injured while riding three-wheeled ATVs.

III. Vertical falls

Falls are common among all age groups. The best predictor of injury is distance fallen, body position, and the surface struck. In general, a fall greater than three times the height of an individual is likely to cause serious injury. Children tend to land on their heads (heaviest part of the body), but adults are more likely to land on feet and hands (especially in falls less than 10 ft). Thus children commonly sustain head injuries and adults commonly get injuries to the extremities. Victims who land on their feet frequently get compression fractures of their lumbar spines. Internal injuries occur frequently if the trunk of the body is the initial impact area. There may be penetrating wounds

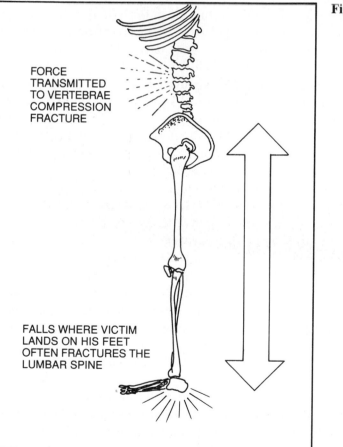

Figure 2–8.

FORCE TRANSMITTED TO VERTEBRAE COMPRESSION FRACTURE

FALLS WHERE VICTIM LANDS ON HIS FEET OFTEN FRACTURES THE LUMBAR SPINE

if protruding objects are present in the surface on which the victim falls. This may present some difficulty since these objects should not be removed, but if at all possible, left in the victim and transported with the victim to the emergency department.

IV. **Projectile penetration**

Many conditions can create projectiles. We are familiar with rifles, pistols, and shotguns, but remember that lawn mowers, circular saws, and other power tools are also capable of producing deadly projectiles.

A. *Firearms*

1. *High-velocity projectiles:* A high-velocity projectile is one traveling greater than 2000 ft per second. This limits this group to hunting and military rifles and a few special-purpose handguns. Bullets from these weapons create tissue damage extending several inches around the path of the bullet. The greatest damage is done to solid organs. Those bullets that deform (hollow point) or tumble in flesh (high velocity–small caliber) create even larger paths of destruction because they transfer all of their energy to the tissue. Large-caliber bullets that go completely through the body without deforming may cause relatively less tissue damage because they do not transfer as much energy to the body. As a practical matter, always assume that any wound made by a hunting or military rifle bullet is worse than it initially appears. This holds true even if the wound appears to be minor. These weapons almost never cause minor wounds. Any wound of an extremity will frequently result in amputation.

2. *Low-velocity projectiles:* These include the bullets fired by most handguns (including magnums) and submachine guns. Most other missiles from lawn mowers and power tools also fall into this group. These missiles create less organ damage because they carry less energy. They are certainly capable of producing fatal wounds if they strike a vital area. The common .22-caliber bullet often causes extensive internal organ damage because it is light and easily deflected inside the body. It often penetrates multiple organs after following an unpredictable path through the body. Knowing the angle of penetration helps to predict organ damage, but never assume that the bullet did not change direction within the body. Even if you find entrance and exit wounds, you cannot be sure the missile followed a straight path between the two points. It is

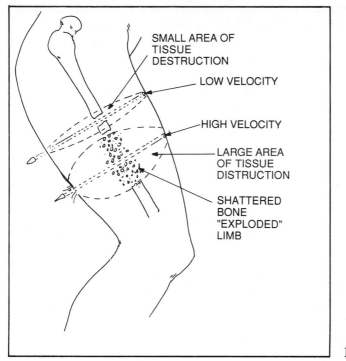

SMALL AREA OF
TISSUE
DESTRUCTION

LOW VELOCITY

HIGH VELOCITY

LARGE AREA
OF TISSUE
DISTRUCTION

SHATTERED
BONE
"EXPLODED"
LIMB

Figure 2-9.

common to have what appears to be a through-and-through head wound that actually turns out to be caused by a small-caliber pistol bullet that enters on one side, slides around the outside of the skull, and exits the scalp on the other side, causing no serious injury. As a practical point, always assume and prepare for the worst with bullet wounds. Do not assume that today's BB guns cannot cause fatal wounds. At close range they will frequently penetrate the skull or chest of a small child.

3. *Shotgun wounds:* The energy imparted depends on the gauge, the size of the pellets, the powder charge, and the distance from the victim. The most frequently encountered injury is from a 12-gauge shotgun firing No. 6 or larger pellets (about BB size). A pattern with a diameter of 6 inches or less indicates concentrated energy from close range. A 12-gauge full-choke shotgun with No. 6 pellets will concentrate 95 percent of the pellets into a 9-inch circle at 10 yards. A shotgun wound from close range (5 to 6 ft) will usually cause massive tissue distruction with associated high mortality rate.

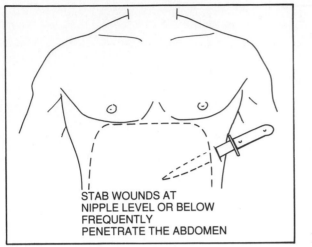

STAB WOUNDS AT
NIPPLE LEVEL OR BELOW
FREQUENTLY
PENETRATE THE ABDOMEN

Figure 2–10.

B. *Knives:* Blade length and angle of penetration are important predictors of injury. If the knife is still in the body, leave it in place. If it is not present, ask the victim or any witnesses to describe the length of the blade, the angle of penetration, and what position the victim's body was in at the time of the stabbing. It is common for abdominal stabs to have penetrated the chest and injured the heart or lungs. Lower chest wounds almost always involve the abdomen since most of the major abdominal organs are under the ribs.

V. **Blast injury**

Explosions are becoming more common in the industrialized world in which we live. There are three mechanisms involved in explosion injuries. The first or primary injury is from the high-pressure blast wave of the explosion. This causes the most damage to air-filled or hollow organs such as the lungs and intestinal tract. Frothy blood from the lungs is the most common presentation. The victim may have fatal injuries with no external signs. Secondary injuries are caused by the debris (rocks, splinters, etc.) thrown by the blast. These usually cause obvious injuries such as cuts, bruises, fractures, and burns. If the victim is blown off his feet by the blast, he will then sustain tertiary injuries or those caused when his body strikes the ground or some other object. These are much the same as to be expected from being ejected from an auto. Both external and internal injuries may occur. Always suspect lung injuries in a blast victim.

Summary

Always attempt to recreate the trauma scene in order to become aware of mechanisms by which injuries may have been produced. Try to answer the following questions:

1. What happened?
2. What sort of force (energy) was applied?
3. To what part of the body and in what direction was the force applied?
4. How much force was involved (speed, mass, voltage)?

It has been said, "An emergency no longer exists when you are prepared to treat it." A knowledge of mechanisms of injury and transfer of energy prepares you for rapid evaluation of obvious injuries, as well as anticipation of potential injuries. Treatment can be one step ahead of problems. This translates into lives being saved.

Chapter 3

INITIAL EVALUATION OF THE TRAUMA VICTIM

It is heartbreaking to see a life lost, especially if it happens because treatment is instituted too little and too late. In the severely injured patient, time is of the essence. Every action in the field must have a lifesaving purpose because you are trading minutes of the "golden hour" for every action done before transport. Evaluation and resuscitation must be reduced to the most efficient and critical steps. The habit of assessing and treating every trauma patient in a preplanned logical and sequential manner must be developed.

There are certain concepts you must always keep in mind when you approach patients who are injured:

1. Trauma patients are not "treated" in the field. They are treated in the emergency department or operating room. Only critical interventions are made in the field.
2. Most trauma fatalities are due to the patient not arriving in the operating room soon enough to be saved.
3. All trauma care revolves around making the most efficient use of time so that the patient is transported to the *appropriate* hospital as soon as possible.

As the first person to treat the patient, you are a *critical* member of the EMS system. The trauma victim's fate depends on the speed, judgment, and skill of your actions.

The "golden hour" begins when the victim is injured, not when you begin your evaluation. Minutes lost before you arrive are just as important as minutes lost because of disorganized actions at the scene. You must learn to squeeze the most out of *every* minute of the rescue process. Rapid management does not mean simply racing down the highway at breakneck speed, throwing the victim into the back of the ambulance, and racing to the nearest emergency department. You can maximize the patient's chance of survival if you perform your duties properly during the six stages of an ambulance call. These are outlined below.

1. *Predispatch:* This is the first (and often ignored) stage of prehospital care. You cannot give lifesaving care if you cannot find the accident, if you do not know the shortest route, or if your ambulance or rescue vehicle is not ready to respond. Before you begin taking ambulance calls, you must learn the area that you serve. You should know the streets and highways well enough to pick the shortest route immediately. You should keep in mind an alternate route in case traffic conditions, weather, or other conditions make it unwise to take the shortest route. Fast driving will not make up for lack of map training. Between runs the vehicle must be checked, fueled, and restocked immediately.

2. *Dispatch:* The rescue crew must have the proper information to respond rapidly to a call:
   a. *Exact nature of the call:* What happened? How many victims? Are there dangers at the scene? Will special equipment be needed?
   b. *Exact location of the call:* This cannot be overemphasized. If an exact address cannot be given, get directions that are as precise as possible.
   c. *Callback number:* This can be invaluable if you have trouble locating the scene of the accident. Units equipped with a radio telephone switch station (RTSS) or cellular telephone can call back for more information about the accident while they are responding.

3. *Travel to the scene:* Make a rapid, yet careful response using your best judgment concerning the fastest route. Obtain the necessary information from the dispatcher (or from a callback to the scene) so you can make decisions about backup help and equipment needed.

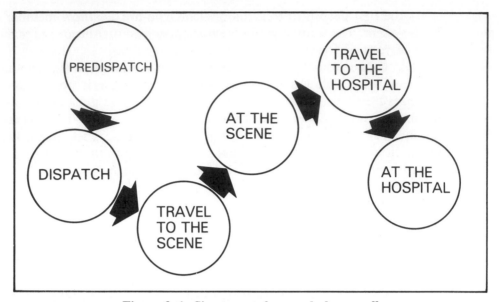

Figure 3–1. Six stages of an ambulance call.

4. *Actions at the scene:* You must make a quick assessment of the overall situation. Park the ambulance as close as possible, keeping in mind the dangers (i.e., traffic, fire, explosion, power lines) of the scene. Quickly note the apparent mechanisms of injury. Be aware of the number of victims and call for help if needed. As a general rule, one ambulance is needed for every seriously injured victim. Begin evaluation of the most seriously injured victim first (unless you have a disaster, in which case use disaster protocols). Evaluate, resuscitate, and package the patients using the priority plan. Be rapid but careful and *gentle.* Rough handling aggravates injuries.

5. *Travel to the hospital:* Select the most suitable route and hospital according to your local protocols. The most experienced EMT should remain at the patient's side and provide continuous monitoring. Notify medical control if the patient's condition deteriorates during transport. Notify the receiving facility of your estimated time of arrival and special needs. It is important to report to medical control as early as possible. Frequently, critical members of the trauma team (surgeons, operating room crew, etc.) must be called to the hospital. Minutes lost waiting on the proper physician to arrive can be just as fatal as minutes lost waiting on the EMT to arrive.

6. *Actions at the hospital:* You should continue your care until you are relieved by the emergency department staff; never leave a patient unattended. Report pertinent information about the victim to the nurse

or physician in charge. This should include a description of the scene, mechanisms of injuries, observed and suspected injuries, procedures performed, and changes in condition. Remain as long as you are needed. When no longer required, you should complete your run report and immediately prepare your vehicle for return to service.

Trauma Assessment

On scene trauma asssessment begins with certain actions *before* you approach the victim. Failure to perform preliminary actions may jeopardize your life as well as your patient.

Preliminary Actions at the Scene

A. *Scene survey*
 1. Assess the scene for hazards.
    a. Is the ambulance or rescue vehicle parked in the nearest safe place?
    b. Is it safe to approach the victim?
    c. Do you need special equipment (turnout gear, breathing equipment) to approach the victim? *Do not become a victim!*
    d. Does the victim require immediate movement because of hazards?
 2. Does the victim require extrication? Is special equipment needed?
 3. Note the mechanisms of injury.
 4. Note the number of victims.
    a. If more than one victim, call for more ambulances now. Usually, one ambulance is needed for each seriously injured victim. If many victims, notify medical control to initiate the disaster protocol.
    b. Are all victims accounted for? If there are no conscious victims, look for schoolbooks or diaper bag in car, passenger list, and similar items.
B. *Equipment:* If possible, carry all essential equipment to the scene as you go. This prevents loss of time running back and forth to the rescue vehicle. You will almost aways need:
 1. Long backboard with attached head immobilization device.
 2. Cervical immobilization device.
 3. Oxygen and airway equipment.
 4. Antishock garment.
 5. Trauma box (bandage material, BP cuff, stethoscope).

Patient Assessment and Management

There are four steps in the management of the trauma victim:

1. *Primary survey:* to find all immediate threats to life
2. *Transport decision and critical interventions:* to decide if a life threat exists ("load and go" situation) and if a lifesaving intervention *must* be done before or during transport
3. *Secondary survey:* to reassess for change and do a rapid, complete head-to-toe exam and communicate these to medical control
4. *Definitive care:* the final stabilization, often requiring surgery and blood, usually taking place in the operating room, and hopefully taking place within the first hour after injury

To make the most efficient use of time, patient assessment is divided into:

1. *Primary survey:* This is a rapid exam to determine life-threatening conditions. The information that you gather here is used to make decisions about critical interventions and time of transport. This exam should not take over $1\frac{1}{2}$ to 2 minutes. This exam is so important that nothing is allowed to interrupt it except airway obstruction or cardiac arrest. Respiratory distress (other than airway obstruction) is not an indication to interrupt the primary survey because the cause of respiratory distress is frequently found during examination of the chest. Major bleeding is also controlled at this time.

2. *Transport decision and critical interventions:* When you finish the primary survey, you have enough information to decide if a critical situation is present. Patients with critical trauma situations are immediately transported. Almost all treatment will be done during transport. Certain interventions will have to be done on the scene (attempt removal of airway obstruction, seal sucking chest wounds, stop major bleeding, hyperventilate, etc.) but most treatment must wait until the patient is in the ambulance and transport is begun. You must spend your patients minutes wisely; the critical patient has none to spare!

3. *Secondary survey:* Critical patients always have this exam done during transport. If the primary survey has revealed no critical condition, you perform this exam on the scene. The secondary survey is a rapid, detailed exam to pick up all injuries, both obvious and potential. This exam also establishes the baseline from which many treatment decisions will eventually be made. It is important to record this exam.

4. *Communications with medical control:* This is a trauma skill that is often performed poorly. Critical patients require early contact with medical control so that the hospital is prepared for your arrival and appropriate surgeons are notified. Most patients are not critical and communications can wait until you are ready to transport. All communications should be concise and to the point.

Assessment Priorities

A. *Primary survey*
  1. Evaluate *Airway,* C-spine control, and initial level of consciousness.
  2. Evaluate *Breathing.*
  3. Evaluate *Circulation.*
  4. Stop major *bleeding.*
B. *Transport decision and critical interventions*
C. *Secondary survey*
  1. Vital signs
  2. History of patient and trauma event
  3. Head-to-toes exam (including neurological)
  4. Further bandaging and splinting
  5. Continual monitoring

These steps must be memorized until you can perform them in the correct sequence without stopping to think about what comes next. They are the ABCs of Basic Trauma Life Support.

Patient Assessment Using the Priority Plan

Once you approach the victim, your exam should proceed quickly and smoothly. Unless held up by extrication, on-scene time should be under 10 minutes. Critical victims should have on scene times of 5 minutes or less. Nothing interrupts the primary survey except treatment of airway obstruction or cardiac arrest.

A. *Evaluate airway, C-spine control, and initial LOC (level of consciousness):* Assessment begins immediately; even if the victim is being extricated. Extrication should not interfere with patient care. The same priorities apply continually before, during, and after extrication. The team leader should approach the victim from the front (face to face, so that he does not turn his head to see you). A second EMT immediately, gently but firmly, stabilizes the neck in a neutral position. He must

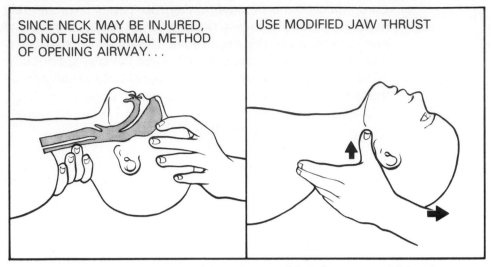

Figure 3–2. Opening airway using modified jaw thrust. Maintain in-line stabilization while pushing up on the angles of the jaw with your thumbs.

not release his hold on the neck until someone relieves him or a suitable stabilization device is applied. The team leader should say to the patient: "We are EMTs here to help you. What happened? The patient's reply gives immediate information about both the airway and the level of consciousness. If the patient responds appropriately to your question, you have established that he has an open airway and his level of consciousness is normal. If the patient cannot speak or is unconscious, you must further evaluate the airway. Look, listen, and feel for movement of air. Open the mouth and clear the airway if necessary. If the airway is obstructed, use the appropriate method to open before finishing the primary survey. Because of the ever-present danger of spinal injury, you must never extend the neck to open the airway of a trauma patient. Patients with airway difficulty or decreased level of consciousness are in the rapid transport category. All patients with decreased LOC should get oxygen and hyperventilation (24 breaths per minute). Your partner may use his knees to maintain immobilization of the neck, freeing his hands to apply oxygen or use a bag-valve–mask to assist ventilation. This is another reason that all equipment should be within immediate reach. If you assist ventilation, be sure that the patient not only gets an adequate ventilatory rate, but also an adequate volume with each breath.

B.   *Assess breathing and circulation:* It is impractical to separate evaluation of breathing and circulation since you must check both as you quickly look, listen, and feel the neck and chest. There is much information to be gained when this examination is performed correctly. (*Remember:* If the patient is not breathing, you must immediately give two full breaths and then check for a carotid pulse. If there is no pulse, you must begin cardiopulmonary resuscitation.) After your partner has immobilized the neck and (if necessary) opened the airway with a modified jaw thrust, you should proceed with evaluation of breathing and circulation in the following manner.

1. Place your face over the patient's mouth so that you can judge both the rate and quality of breathing. Is breathing too fast (> 24 per minute) or too slow (< 12 per minute)? Is the victim moving an adequate volume of air when he breathes? Any abnormality of breathing signals a search for the cause as well as administration of oxygen and possibly breathing assistance. Your partner can apply the nonrebreather oxygen mask or bag–valve device without interrupting your survey.

2. As your partner holds the neck stable, he will find that it is simple to feel the carotid pulse with his index finger. He should note rate and quality, then compare with your evaluation of the pulse at the wrist. Also evaluate skin color/condition and capillary refill. This information, combined with LOC, is the best early assessment of circulatory status and the presence of shock. If the pulse is present at the neck and the wrist, the blood pressure is greater than 80 mmHg (it may be normal—judge by the strength of the pulse—it is not yet time to use the blood pressure cuff). If the pulse is present at the neck but not at the wrist, the blood pressure is between 60 and 80 mmHg. This means *late* shock. Even if the pulse is present and strong at the neck and wrist, you may be able to diagnose *early* shock by other signs. Other signs of shock include slow capillary refill, rapid heart rate (> 100 per minute), cold sweaty skin, pale appearance, confusion, weakness, or thirst. *Remember:* The patient with spinal shock may not be pale, cold, or sweaty and will not have a rapid pulse. He will have a low blood pressure and paralysis. All patients with shock should get oxygen and should have the antishock garment applied as soon as they are on the backboard.

3. As soon as you have noted the breathing and pulse, quickly look and feel to determine if the trachea is in the midline, if the neck veins are flat or distended, and if there is discoloration or swelling. You may apply a rigid extrication collar at this time.

4. Now look, feel, and listen to the chest. If there is any difficulty with respiration, the chest must be bared for examination: This

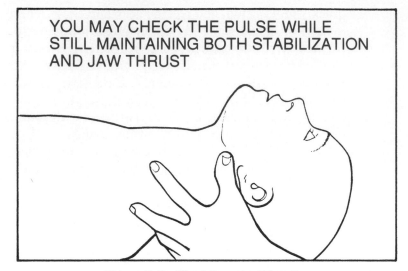

YOU MAY CHECK THE PULSE WHILE
STILL MAINTAINING BOTH STABILIZATION
AND JAW THRUST

Figure 3–3. Checking carotid pulse.

is no time for modesty; chest injuries often kill quickly. Look for sucking chest wounds, flail segments, contusions, or deformities. Note if the ribs rise with respiration or if there is only diaphragmatic breathing. Feel for instability, tenderness, or crepitation. Listen for breath sounds. Are they *present and equal* on both sides? If breath sounds are not equal (decreased or absent on one side), you should determine if tension pneumothorax is present. If abnormalities are found here (open chest wound, flail chest, respiratory difficulty), you should make the appropriate intervention (seal open wound, *hand stabilize* flail, give oxygen, assist ventilation).

5. *Stop active bleeding:* Your other partner should have already done this, or at least begun to do this. Almost all bleeding can be stopped by direct pressure; use gauze pads and bandage or elastic wraps. You may use air splints or antishock garment to tamponade bleeding. Tourniquets may be needed in *rare* situations. If a dressing becomes blood soaked, you may remove the dressing and redress once to be sure that you are applying pressure to the bleeding site. It is important that you report such excessive bleeding to the receiving physician. Do not use clamps to stop bleeders; you may cause injuries to other structures (nerves are present alongside arteries).

6. *Conduct MAST survey:* If your primary survey identified a critical trauma situation, you should modify the primary survey by adding the MAST survey. Since a critical condition requires transport before performing the secondary survey, and you will frequently have to apply the antishock garment (MAST,PASG) before you do the secondary survey, you need to check quickly the areas of the body that will be hidden by the garment. You must expose the body to do this. Quickly cut off clothes, maintaining body warmth and modesty with a sheet or blanket. The MAST survey consists of quickly examining the abdomen, pelvis and legs.

At this point you have enough information to determine critical trauma situations that should be treated by "load and go."

Critical Injuries/Conditions

A. *Airway obstruction unrelieved by mechanical methods* (i.e., suction, forceps)
B. *Conditions resulting in possible inadequate breathing*
   1. Large open chest wound (sucking chest wound)
   2. Large flail chest
   3. Tension pneumothorax
   4. Major thoracic airway injury
C. *Traumatic cardiopulmonary arrest*
D. *Shock*
   1. Hemorrhagic
   2. Spinal
   3. Myocardial contusion
   4. Pericardial tamponade
E. *Head injury with decreased level of consciousness*

This can be further simplified into three conditions based on signs and symptoms:

1. *Difficulty with respiration*
2. *Difficulty with circulation (shock)*
3. *Decreased level of consciousness*

Any trauma patient with one or more of these conditions falls into the "load and go" category. When you finish the primary survey, you have enough information to decide if the patient is critical or stable. If the patient has one of the critical conditions, you should immediately transfer him to a long backboard (check his back as you log-roll him), apply MAST and oxygen, load him into an ambulance (if available), and transport rapidly to the nearest appropriate emergency facility. Lifesaving procedures may be needed but should not hold up transport. There are a few brief procedures that are done while at the scene (attempt to relieve airway obstruction, seal sucking chest wound, hand stabilize flail, hyperventilate, begin CPR), but most are reserved for transport. You must weigh every field procedure against the time it will take to perform. You are spending minutes of the patient's golden hour; be sure the procedure is worth the cost. Nonlifesaving procedures (splinting and bandaging) must not hold up transport. Be sure to call medical control early so that the hospital is prepared for your arrival.

If the primary survey fails to identify a critical trauma situation, you should transfer the victim to the backboard (check the back) and proceed with the secondary survey.

Secondary Survey

This exam is to provide a rapid, orderly head-to-toes survey to assess for other injuries. The critical patient has this exam performed during transport to the hospital. The patient who appears stable should have this exam done at the scene. Even if the patient appears stable and you elect to perform this exam at the scene, keep the time under 5 minutes. "Stable" patients may become "unstable" quite rapidly.

1. Check vital signs. Record pulse, respiration, and blood pressure (obtain accurate recordings and use the BP cuff now).
2. Obtain a history of the injury (your partner may already have done this).
   a. Personal observation.
   b. Bystanders.
   c. Victim. Look for a Medic Alert tag in unconscious patients. Take an AMPLE history from conscious patients:
      A   allergies
      M   medications
      P   past medical history (other illnesses)
      L   last meal (when was it eaten)
      E   events preceding the accident
3. Do a head-to-toes exam.

a. Begin at the head examining for contusions, lacerations, raccoon eyes, Battle's sign, and drainage of blood or fluid from the ears or nose. Assess the airway again.

b. Check the neck again. Look for lacerations, contusions, tenderness, distended neck veins, or deviated trachea. Check the pulse again. If not already done, apply a cervical immobilization device at this time.

c. Recheck the chest. Be sure that breath sounds are still present and equal on each side. Recheck seals over open wounds. Be sure that flails are well stabilized (hand stabilization is adequate until you are in the ambulance).

d. Examine the abdomen. Look for signs of blunt or penetrating trauma. Feel for tenderness. Do not waste time listening for bowel sounds. If the abdomen is painful to gentle pressure during examination, you can expect the patient to be bleeding internally. If the abdomen is both distended and painful, you can expect hemorrhagic shock very quickly.

e. Assess pelvis and extremities. Be sure to check and record distal sensation and pulses on all fractures. Do this before and after straightening any fracture. Angulated fractures of the upper extremities are usually best splinted as found. Most fractures of the lower extremities are straightened by using traction splints or air splints. *Critical patients have all splints applied during transport.*

Transport immediately if your secondary survey reveals any of the following:

1. Tender, distended abdomen
2. Pelvic instability
3. Bilateral femur fractures

Even though the patient may appear stable at this time, he will probably soon develop shock because of the large blood loss that is associated with these injuries.

4. Do a brief neurological exam. The neurological exam is very simple, but is frequently forgotten. It gives important baseline information that is used in later treatment decisions. Perform and record this exam.
   a. *Level of consciousness*
      A alert
      V responds to verbal stimuli
      P responds to pain
      U unresponsive

b. *Motor:* Can he move fingers and toes?
c. *Sensation:* Can he feel you when you touch his fingers and toes? Does the unconscious patient respond when you pinch his fingers and toes?
d. *Pupils:* Are they equal or unequal? Do they respond to light?

5. If necessary, finish bandaging and splinting.
6. Continually monitor and reevaluate the patient.
   If the patient's condition worsens, repeat the primary survey: EVERY STEP.
   Accurately record what you see and what you do. Record changes in the patient's condition during transport. Record the time the antishock garment or tourniquet is applied. Extenuating circumstances or significant details should be recorded in the comments or remarks section of the run report.

Contacting Medical Control

This is important so that the emergency department can be prepared for the arrival of the patient. It is extremely important to do this as early as possible when you have a patient with a critical condition. It takes time to get the appropriate surgeon and the operating room team called in. The critical victim has no time to wait. Following is the procedure to communicate with medical control:

1. Identify yourself; give level of training and organization.
2. Give the patient's approximate age, sex, mechanism of injuries, nature of the injuries, vital signs, level of consciousness, procedures performed, and the patient's response.
3. Transport the patient to the facility named by medical control.
4. Notify the facility of the estimated time of arrival (ETA), the condition of the patient, and any special needs on arrival.

Summary

This is the content of the course in one chapter: a rapid, orderly, thorough examination of the trauma patient with priorities of examination and treatment always in mind. The continuous practice of approaching the patient in this way will allow you to concentrate on the patient rather than trying to figure out what to do next. Optimum speed is achieved by teamwork. Teamwork is achieved by practice. During the predispatch stage, you should plan regular exercises in patient evaluation in order to perfect each team member's role in the priority plan. The following pages contain a brief outline of the primary and secondary survey as well as the thoughts that should go through your mind as you perform the survey.

THE BASIC TRAUMA LIFE SUPPORT PRIMARY SURVEY

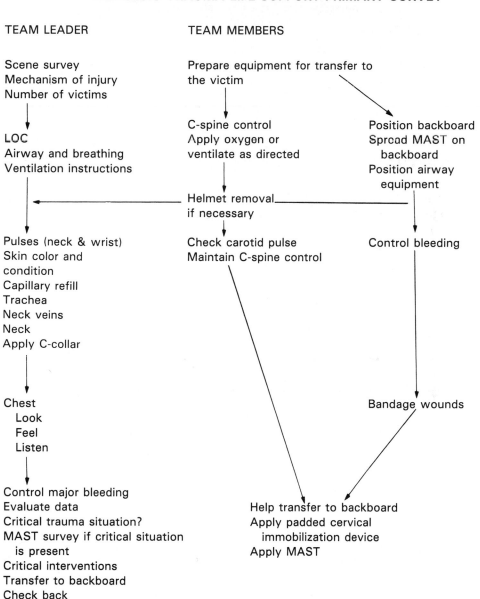

TEAM LEADER

TEAM MEMBERS

Scene survey
Mechanism of injury
Number of victims

Prepare equipment for transfer to
the victim

LOC
Airway and breathing
Ventilation instructions

C-spine control
Apply oxygen or
ventilate as directed

Position backboard
Spread MAST on
backboard
Position airway
equipment

Helmet removal
if necessary

Pulses (neck & wrist)
Skin color and
condition
Capillary refill
Trachea
Neck veins
Neck
Apply C-collar

Check carotid pulse
Maintain C-spine control

Control bleeding

Chest
　Look
　Feel
　Listen

Bandage wounds

Control major bleeding
Evaluate data
Critical trauma situation?
MAST survey if critical situation
　is present
Critical interventions
Transfer to backboard
Check back

Help transfer to backboard
Apply padded cervical
　immobilization device
Apply MAST

PARROT PHRASES

This is what should be going through your mind as you perform each step of the survey. They are also the phrases you should repeat (like a parrot) to the instructor as you are being tested on patient evaluation.

SCENE SURVEY

I am surveying the scene. Are there any dangers?
I am surveying for mechanisms of injury.
Are there any other victims?

LEVEL OF CONSCIOUSNESS

We are EMTs here to help you. What happened?
Please do not move until we have checked you for injuries.

AIRWAY

Is the airway clear?
What is the rate and quality of respiration?

VENTILATION INSTRUCTIONS

Order oxygen for any airway difficulty, head injury, or shock.
Assist ventilation if hypoventilating.
Hyperventilate altered level of consciousness.

PULSES

What is the rate and quality of the pulse at the neck and the wrist?

SKIN COLOR AND CONDITION

What is the skin color and condition?

CAPILLARY REFILL

Is the capillary refill normal or delayed?

TRACHEA

Is the trachea midline or deviated?

NECK VEINS

Are the neck veins flat or distended?

NECK

Are there signs of trauma to the neck?

CHEST

I am looking at the chest. Are there any penetrations, contusions, deformities, or paradoxical motions?

I am feeling of the chest. Is there any crepitation, tenderness, or instability?

I am listening to the chest. Are the breath sounds present and equal?

If breath sounds are not equal:

I am percussing the chest. Is there tympany (hyperresonance) or dullness on either side?

BLEEDING

Is there any obvious external bleeding?

MAST SURVEY
ABDOMEN

Are there any contusions, penetrations, distention, or tenderness of the abdomen?

PELVIS

Is the pelvis tender or unstable?

LOWER EXTREMITIES

Is there any sign of trauma to the legs?

EXAM OF THE BACK
(Done during transfer to the backboard)

Is there any sign of trauma to the back?

THE BASIC TRAUMA LIFE SUPPORT SECONDARY SURVEY

When performing the secondary survey, you must visualize and palpate from head to toes. Everyone gets a secondary survey: stable patients while at the scene, critical patients during transport. If other team members are available, the blood pressure and accurate pulse and respiratory rates may be taken by one of them.

HEAD

1. Palpate
   Entire scalp for lacerations or contusions
   Face for tenderness or fractures
2. Look
   For Battle's sign
   For blood or fluid in ears
   For raccoon eyes
   For blood or fluid from nose
   For pupillary size, equality, reaction to light
   For burns of face, nose hairs, mouth
   For skin changes
       Pallor
       Cyanosis
       Diaphoresis
       Bruising
3. Reassess
   a. Airway
      Check for carbonacious (sooty) sputum if burn victim
   b. Breathing
      Rate (accurately and record)
      Quality
   c. Circulation
      Rate (accurately and record)
      Quality
      Blood pressure (done by partner if possible)

NECK (If collar has been applied, remove the front)

Signs of trauma?
JVD?
Tracheal deviation?

CHEST

Look for penetrations, contusions, deformities, or paradoxical motions
Feel for instability, tenderness, crepitation
Listen for breath sounds in all lung fields
Percuss if breath sounds unequal

ABDOMEN (If MAST has been applied, this has been completed)

Look for penetrations, contusions, distention
Palpate all four quadrants for tenderness

PELVIS (If MAST has been applied, this has been completed)

Compress laterally and over symphysis for tenderness or instability

LOWER EXTREMITIES (If MAST applied, do pulses, neuro, cap refill)

Visualize and palpate for signs of trauma
Check distal pulses
Do neurological
                 sensory (pinch toes)
                 motor (have patient move toes)
Check range of motion
Repeat capillary refill (unless you have already made the diagnosis of shock)

UPPER EXTREMITIES

Visualize and palpate for signs of trauma
Begin at the midline, checking clavicles, shoulders, arms, and hands
Check distal pulses
Do neurological
    sensory (pinch fingers)
    motor (have patient move fingers)
Check range of motion
Repeat capillary refill (unless you have already made the diagnosis of shock)

PARROT PHRASES: SECONDARY SURVEY

HEAD

I am feeling the scalp: Are there lacerations, contusions, or deformity?
I am feeling the face: Are there contusions or deformity?
Are Battle's sign or raccoon eyes present?
Is there blood or fluid draining from the ears or nose?
What is pupillary size? Are they equal? Do they react to light?
Is there pallor, cyanosis, diaphoresis, or bruising?
Are there burns of the face, nose hairs, or inside the mouth?

AIRWAY

Is the airway clear?
What is the rate and quality of respiration?
Is there soot in the sputum (if a burn victim)?

CIRCULATION

What is the rate and quality of the pulse?
What is the blood pressure?
What is skin color and condition?
Is the capillary refill normal or delayed? (Not done if diagnosis of shock is already made)

NECK

Are there signs of trauma to the neck?
Are the neck veins flat or distended?
Is the trachea midline or deviated?

CHEST

I am looking at the chest. Are there any penetrations, contusions, deformities, or paradoxical motion?
I am feeling the chest. Is there any crepitation, tenderness, or instability?
I am listening to the chest. Are the breath sounds present and equal?
I am percussing the chest. Is it hyperresonant or dull? (Do only if breath sounds are unequal)

UPPER EXTREMITIES

Is there any sign of trauma to the arms?
Are pulses present?
Can he feel me touch his fingers?
Can he move his fingers?
Is range of motion normal?
Is capillary refill normal or delayed? (Not done if diagnosis of shock has already been made)

ABDOMEN (If MAST has been applied, this has been completed)

I am looking at the abdomen. Are there penetrations, contusions, or distention?
I am feeling the abdomen. Is there any tenderness?

PELVIS (If MAST has been applied, this has been completed)

Is the pelvis tender or unstable?

LOWER EXTREMITIES (If MAST has been applied, do pulses, neuro, and capillary refill)

Are there any signs of trauma to the legs?
Are pulses present?
Can he feel me touch his toes?
Can he move his toes?
Is range of motion normal?
Is capillary refill normal or delayed? (Not done if diagnosis of shock has already been made)

RAPID PATIENT ASSESSMENT
I.   Scene survey
II.   Carry all essential equipment as you approach the victim
III.   Evaluate the victim

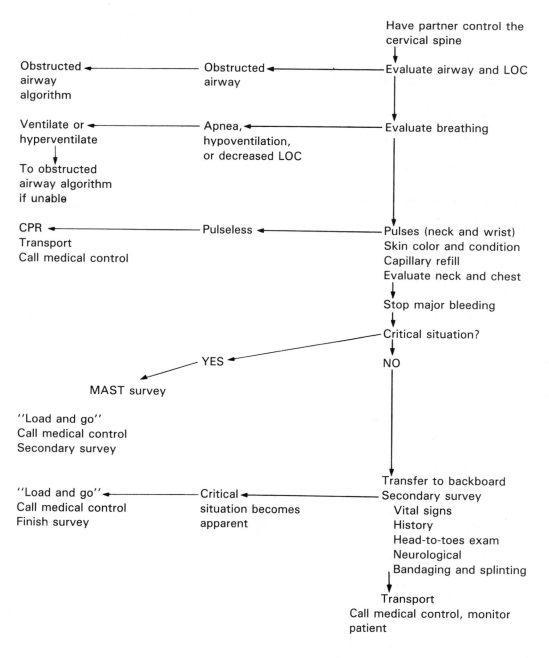

Have partner control the
cervical spine

Obstructed ◄————————— Obstructed ◄———————— Evaluate airway and LOC
airway   airway
algorithm

Ventilate or ◄———————— Apnea, ◄———————— Evaluate breathing
hyperventilate   hypoventilation,
                            or decreased LOC
To obstructed
airway algorithm
if unable

CPR ◄————————————— Pulseless ◄——————— Pulses (neck and wrist)
Transport   Skin color and condition
Call medical control   Capillary refill
                                             Evaluate neck and chest

                                             Stop major bleeding

                                             Critical situation?

                    YES ◄   NO

          MAST survey

"Load and go"
Call medical control
Secondary survey

                                             Transfer to backboard
"Load and go" ◄——————— Critical ◄————— Secondary survey
Call medical control   situation becomes   Vital signs
Finish survey   apparent   History
                                                      Head-to-toes exam
                                                      Neurological
                                                      Bandaging and splinting

                                             Transport
                                             Call medical control, monitor
                                             patient

OBSTRUCTED AIRWAY ALGORITHM

Examine airway

No respiration

Open airway (jaw thrust or chin lift)

Attempt ventilation

Airway obstructed

Repeat opening maneuver

Attempt ventilation

Remains obstructed

Clear pharynx ─────────────► Airway cleared

(suction, digital removal)

Remains obstructed

Immediately "load and go"

Continue to attempt to
clear the airway and ventilate
(may use chest thrusts)

One team member
inserts oral or NP
airway and hyper-
ventilates with
high-flow oxygen ──────────► "Load and go"

One team member
completes
primary survey

Notify medical control of
critical situation
Adapted from *An Algorithm for Rapid Assessment of the Airway* by
Daniel L. Cavallaro and Patricia J. Mominee

Chapter 4

MANAGING THE AIRWAY

I. **Airway Management in perspective**

The airway is the first priority in the evaluation of any sick or injured patient; if the patient is unable to exchange air, all other efforts at resuscitation are futile. The basic EMT has limited airway management techniques at his disposal, therefore he must perform them perfectly. Basic procedures, aggressively and properly performed, will be adequate airway management in the vast majority of multiple trauma victims.

II. **Anatomy of the Airway (see figure 4.1)**

Air enters the nostrils and/or mouth, passes through the nasopharynx and oropharynx, through the vocal cords (glottic opening) into the trachea and bronchi to the bronchioles, arriving finally at the alveoli where oxygenation of the blood occurs. The key point at which obstruction can occur is the glottic opening just below the epiglottis at the base of the tongue.

III. **Obstruction to Upper Airway**

    A. Tongue: This is the most common obstruction to the airway in an unconscious patient. The tongue attaches to the front of the jaw. One does not "stick one's tongue out, but rather it is pulled out of the mouth by contraction of the genioglossus muscle. When

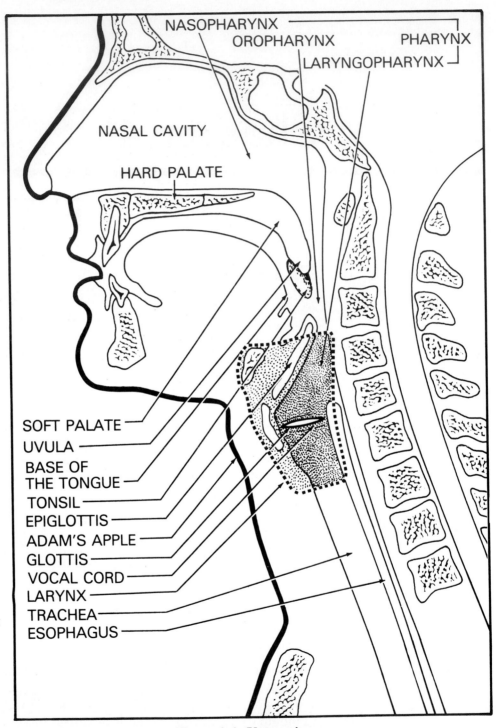

Figure 4–1. Upper airway.

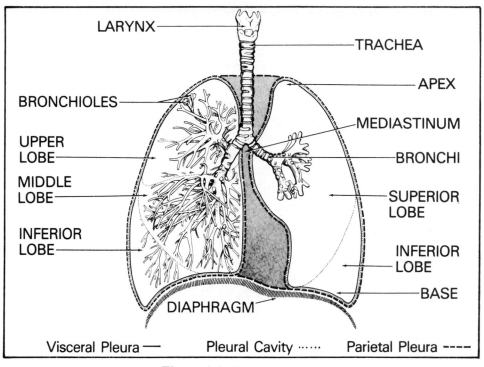

LARYNX

TRACHEA

APEX

BRONCHIOLES

MEDIASTINUM

UPPER
LOBE

BRONCHI

MIDDLE
LOBE

SUPERIOR
LOBE

INFERIOR
LOBE

INFERIOR
LOBE

BASE

DIAPHRAGM

Visceral Pleura —   Pleural Cavity ……   Parietal Pleura ----

Figure 4–2. Lower airways.

unconscious, the slack muscles allow the tongue to fall back in the mouth and obstruct the airway. Since the tongue is attached to the jaw, lifting the jaw has the same effect as contracting the muscles; it it pulls the tongue up and out of the pharynx.

B. *Foreign bodies:* These include vomitus, blood, food, and dentures, among others. As you evaluate for an open airway, always clear the mouth and pharnyx of these foreign bodies using your fingers or suction. You may not be able to remove blood or thick vomitus with suction; in this case, the victim must be log-rolled (stabilize the neck while doing this) into a face-down position to prevent aspiration and to allow gravity to help clear the upper airway.

C. *Edema (swelling):* This includes swelling of the soft tissue of the throat as well as swelling of the vocal cords themselves. Direct injury to the soft tissue of the neck can cause rapid obstruction of the airway by swelling. This presents with stridor similar to epiglottitis, croup, and allergic edema of the vocal cords. A high-pitched or "seal bark" cough is an indication for oxygen and *rapid* transport.

IV. **Techniques for opening the airway**

A. *Manual techniques to open the airway:* Note that the basic cardiac life support (BCLS) method of tilting the head to open the airway is not performed on the trauma victim. If there is any chance of neck injury, one of the following techniques should be used.

1. *Jaw thrust—modified:* This is the method of choice for the trauma victim since it is the only one you can perform while also stabilizing the neck. The other methods require two rescuers. When you place your hands on either side of the neck to stabilize, use your thumbs to push up on the angles of the jaw to open the airway. From this position you can also use your index fingers to check for a carotid pulse.

2. *Chin lift:* This requires two rescuers—one to stabilize the neck and the other to open the airway. The rescuer opening the airway uses his thumb to grasp the chin just below the lower lip while the fingers of that hand are placed underneath the anterior jaw and the chin is gently lifted. The chin lift can be used in connection with mouth-to-mouth breathing.

3. *Jaw lift:* This is the same as the chin lift except that the thumb goes inside the mouth and grasps the lower incisors to lift the jaw. The disadvantages are as follows:

    a. You cannot do mouth-to-mouth breathing.
    b. Wet teeth are slippery.
    c. You may get bitten if the patient regains consciousness or has a seizure.

Figure 4–3. Modified jaw thrust.

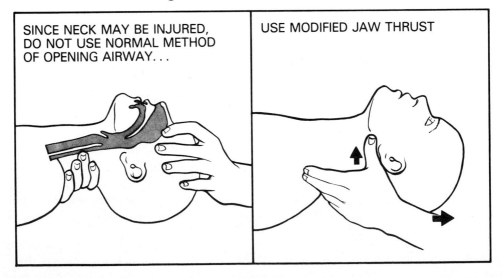

SINCE NECK MAY BE INJURED, DO NOT USE NORMAL METHOD OF OPENING AIRWAY...

USE MODIFIED JAW THRUST

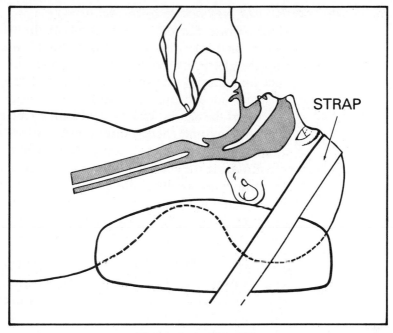

Figure 4–4. Chin lift.

Figure 4–5. Jaw lift.

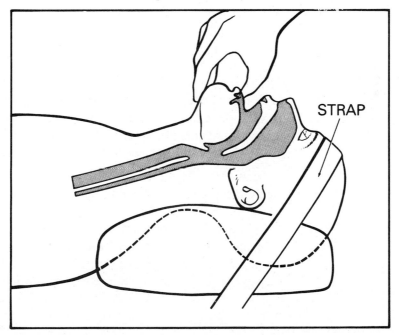

B.   *Mechanical methods to open the airway*
1.   *Oral airway:* The oral airway is a semicircular apparatus of plastic or rubber. Its function is to hold the tongue forward and thus keep the airway open. Because of its shape, incorrect insertion can push the base of the tongue down and obstruct the airway. There are two methods of insertion:
   a.   Insert the airway upside down until it reaches the posterior pharynx and then rotate it 180 degrees so that it slips behind the tongue. Children have a smaller oral cavity. Rotating the curved airway may injure a child's pharynx and cause swelling that may obstruct the airway.
   b.   A better method is to push the tongue out of the way with a tongue blade so that you can insert the oral airway directly into the correct place.

Remember: The oral airway is reserved for use in the unconscious patient with no gag reflex. The use of an oral airway in a patient with an intact gag reflex will cause vomiting.

2.   *Nasopharyngeal airway:* This is a soft rubber or plastic tube about 6 inches in length. This device is tolerated by the conscious patient, but the opening is usually too small to pass a suction catheter. To insert the nasopharyngeal airway, first lubricate well, preferably with a lubricant that contains a local anesthetic. Insert the nasopharyngeal airway through one nostril into the posterior pharynx behind the tongue. The bevel goes toward the nasal septum. You will notice that the airway is made to go into the right nostril. In about 10 to 15 percent of the population, the septum is deviated so that you may not be able to insert the airway into the right nostril. To insert through the left nostril, turn the airway upside down so that the bevel is toward the septum, then insert the airway straight back through the nostril until you reach the posterior pharynx. At this point turn the airway over 180 degrees and insert down the pharynx until it lies behind the tongue.

Remember: The opening through the nasal cavity goes straight back to the pharynx. It does not go upward. Never try to force the airway, you will cause a nosebleed.

All unconscious victims must have constant attention to be sure their airway does not become obstructed. If they have no gag reflex, you should insert an oral or nasopharyngeal airway. If their gag reflex is present (gag when you attempt

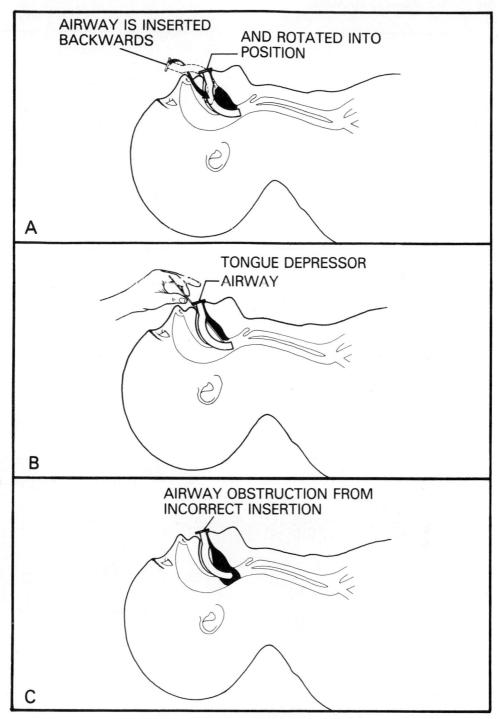

Figure 4–6. Insertion of oral airway.

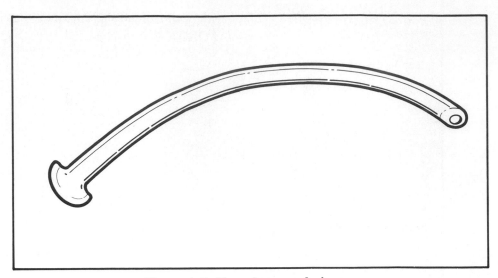

Figure 4–7. Nasopharyngeal airway.

Figure 4–8. Insertion of nasopharyngeal airway into right nostril.

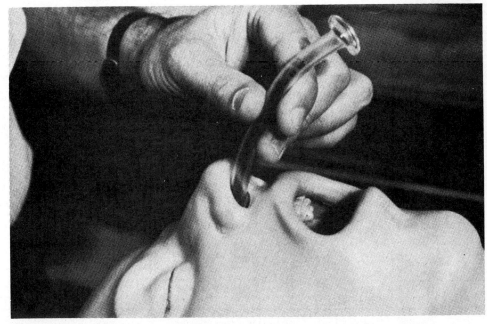

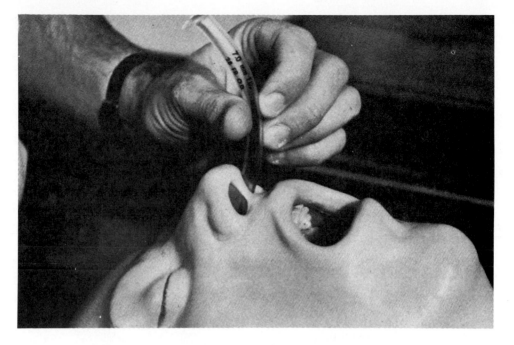

Figure 4–9a. Insertion of nasopharyngeal airway into left nostril. Insert upside down so bevel is toward the septum.

Figure 4–9b. When tip is to the back of the pharynx, rotate airway 180 degrees.

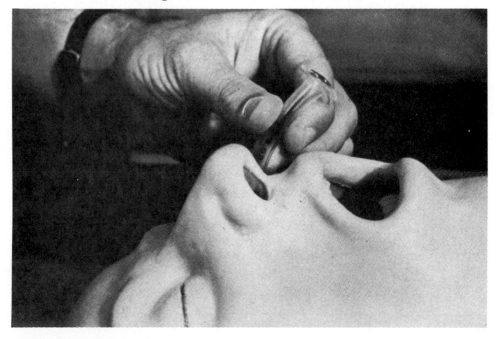

to insert oral airway), you should insert a nasopharyngeal airway and also provide suction as needed to keep the airway open. When strapped onto a backboard, the conscious patient cannot protect his airway. It is your responsibility to prevent aspiration.

V. **Suctioning**

Unconscious trauma victims usually require suctioning to keep the airway from becoming blocked by secretions, vomitus, or blood. There are several good portable suction devices available. You must familiarize yourself with the operation of such equipment before you use it in rescue operations. Often when the victim needs suctioning you have only a few seconds to accomplish this task. Suction equipment must be kept instantly available for use. If your patient vomits, you must be able immediately to lay your hands on the suction. Rapid evaluation and transport means nothing if you neglect this small detail and your patient aspirates. The main complication of suctioning is hypoxia. Remember, while you are suctioning, the victim is getting no oxygen. Vomiting and nosebleed (nasal suctioning) are other complications of suctioning.

VI. **Breathing—ventilation**

A. *Mouth-to-mouth*

1. This is often the superior method of ventilation because of the following:

    a. You can give a larger volume of air with each breath than with a bag–valve device.

    b. You can feel the amount of resistance in the airway.

    c. You can get a better seal on the mouth than with a face mask.

    d. It can be done adequately by one rescuer.

2. The disadvantages of mouth-to-mouth ventilation are as follows:

    a. The face is often covered with blood or vomitus. It takes extreme dedication to do mouth-to-mouth under these circumstances.

    b. It is difficult to give oxygen-enriched air mixtures. You can hold an oxygen line next to your mouth, but this does not provide a large increase over room air.

    c. This is a tiring procedure, and you can hyperventilate if you continue too long.

    d. There is a slight risk of communicable disease with this procedure.

B. *Mouth-to-mask:* The pocket mask is a very useful device that can be used to prevent direct contact of your mouth with the patient's mouth and nose. You can ventilate well as long as you maintain a good seal on the patient's face. This device has a nipple to which an oxygen line can be attached, so you can give oxygen while ventilating. Room air is 21 percent oxygen; by using a pocket mask with oxygen attached and delivering at a rate of 12 liters/min you can give the victim 50 percent oxygen while doing mouth-to-mask ventilation. The mask is best used in conjunction with an oropharyngeal airway to keep the airway open. Hold the mask firmly on the face by placing your thumbs on the side of the mask and grasping the lower jaw with the index, middle, and ring fingers. You should hold the jaw at the angle just below the earlobes; pull upward to open the airway. Ventilate through the opening of the mask. It is easier for inexperienced personnel to ventilate well with this device than with the bag–valve mask.

C. *Bag–valve devices:* These devices are self-inflating and can deliver room air (21 percent oxygen) or an oxygen-enriched air mixture to the patient by way of face mask, EGTA, or ET tube. If a face

Figure 4–10. Pocket mask.

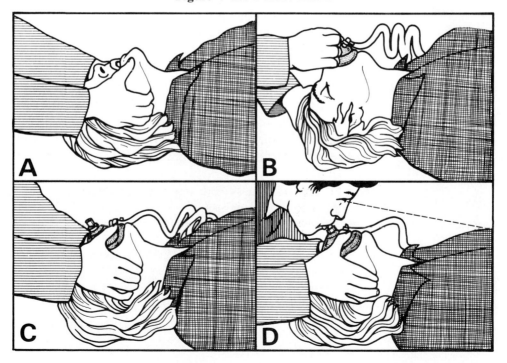

mask is used, it should be used with an oropharyngeal airway to keep the airway open. If oxygen is available, a flow rate of 12 liters/min will increase oxygen concentration to about 40 percent. By the addition of a reservoir bag, the oxygen concentration can be effectively doubled to 80 or 90 percent. All resuscitation bag–valve devices should have an oxygen reservoir attached. A disadvantage of the use of bag–valve devices is that the tidal volume (volume of air delivered) is limited by the size of the bag, the size of your hand, and the seal of the mask on the face. The tidal volume is almost always less than with mouth ventilation. This is partially offset by the increased concentration of oxygen that can be delivered with the bag system. Another major disadvantage is that usually two rescuers are needed to ventilate adequately. One must seal the mask on the face while the other squeezes the bag to ventilate.

D. *Oxygen-powered breathing devices:* Manually triggered devices are in general use and operate on compressed oxygen. They attach to a face mask, EGTA, or ET tube. When a button is pushed, high-flow oxygen that expands the chest is delivered. You cannot feel lung compliance as accurately with this method as you can with mouth or bag ventilation. These devices cause excessive pressure and are notorious for causing gastric distension. Since the trauma patient often has an injury to his chest, any excessive pressure may cause or worsen a tension pneumothorax. These devices should *not* be used in the trauma victim.

E. *Spontaneously breathing patient:* Many trauma victims who are breathing spontaneously should receive oxygen-enriched air. Examples include those patients with carbon monoxide poisoning, smoke inhalation, chest injuries, head injuries, or shock. There are several methods for accomplishing this:

Figure 4–11. Bag-valve mask with reservoir bag attached.

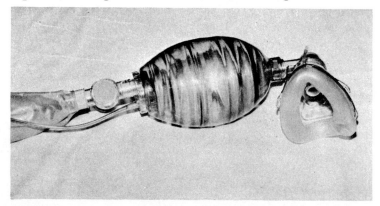

1. *Plastic face mask:* This is usually well tolerated, but some patients cannot stand a face mask because they feel they are smothering. If you use a face mask, give oxygen at a rate of 12 liters/min, which will deliver about 50 percent oxygen.

2. *Face mask with reservoir bag (nonrebreathing mask):* This mask has a reservoir bag attached that acts like the reservoir bag on the bag–valve mask—it essentially doubles the concentration of oxygen (60 to 90 percent, depending on the seal) to the victim. This is the preferred method of giving oxygen.

3. *Nasal cannulas:* These are usually well tolerated by everyone. When set at an oxygen rate of 6 liters/min, they will deliver 25 to 40 percent oxygen.

4. There are other, more sophisticated mask systems available, but limited room in the rescue vehicle dictates that equipment should be kept as simple as possible.

F. *General rules on administration of oxygen to trauma victims*

1. Never withhold oxygen from any patient who is short of breath, has a head injury, or is in shock.

2. Restlessness is a sign of hypoxia; give a restless patient oxygen and look for a cause of shock.

3. Trauma victims who have chronic lung disease are much more likely to need oxygen than is the average victim. Do not withhold it from them. Because of the danger that they may "forget" to breathe while on oxygen, you should remain in attendance to remind them to breathe or assist them in breathing. Use the same oxygen flow rates (6 liters/min nasal cannula, 12 liters/min everything else) as for other victims. The old rule about giving low-flow oxygen to chronic lung disease patients comes from hospital experience, where people often go for hours without being seen by an attendant. This does not hold true in the prehospital setting, where you are constantly monitoring the patient. The flow rate can be adjusted downward after the patient gets to the hospital and arterial blood gases are checked.

4. Trauma victims with a respiratory rate less than 12 per minute are hypoventilating and need oxygen and ventilatory assistance.

5. Trauma victims with a respiratory rate greater than 24 per minute may have acidosis and/or hypoxia or may be hyperventilating from excitement. There is no way to be sure in the prehospital setting, so give all these people oxygen.

6. Oxygen flow rates must be kept simple if you are to remember them in the field. A setting of 12 liters/min will work best with any device (face mask, bag–valve mask) except nasal cannulas. Anything over 6 liters/min is wasted when using nasal cannulas.

AIRWAY
CONSCIOUS PATIENT

Stabilize neck
|
LOC (alert)
|
Note airway
Note rate and quality of respiration

Normal	Abnormal rate or quality	Partial obstruction (stridor)
Continue primary survey	Neck exam	Check for foreign body Examine neck for trauma

One EMT begins high-flow oxygen and assists respiration if needed

One EMT finishes primary survey

"Load and go"

SPECIAL CASES:
1. Profuse bleeding of upper airway.
   High-flow oxygen.
   Constant suction.
   Immediate transport with immediate call to medical control.
   If unable to achieve adequate control with suction, position patient prone (face down) to allow gravity to assist in draining blood away from airway. Use careful C-spine control.

2. Prone victim
   Stabilize neck–LOC–airway.
   If patient is not breathing, log-roll immediately onto backboard. If backboard is not ready, you must log-roll and transfer to backboard after the airway is managed. Go to airway algorithm.

   If patient is breathing, position backboard and log-roll patient onto the backboard. Go to airway algorithm.

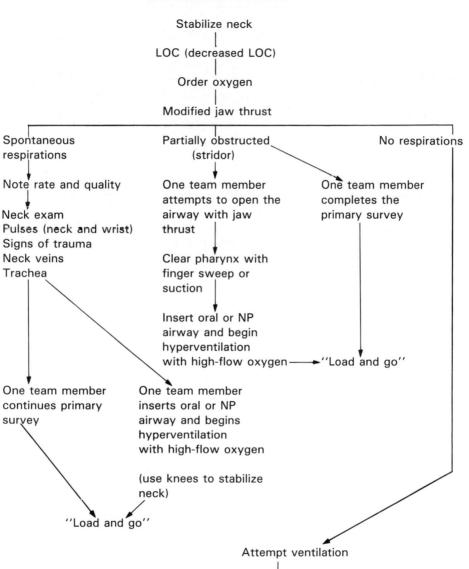

AIRWAY
UNCONSCIOUS PATIENT

Stabilize neck

LOC (decreased LOC)

Order oxygen

Modified jaw thrust

Spontaneous
respirations

Partially obstructed
(stridor)

No respirations

Note rate and quality

Neck exam
Pulses (neck and wrist)
Signs of trauma
Neck veins
Trachea

One team member
attempts to open the
airway with jaw
thrust

Clear pharynx with
finger sweep or
suction

Insert oral or NP
airway and begin
hyperventilation
with high-flow oxygen ——▸ ''Load and go''

One team member
completes the
primary survey

One team member
continues primary
survey

One team member
inserts oral or NP
airway and begins
hyperventilation
with high-flow oxygen

(use knees to stabilize
neck)

''Load and go''

Attempt ventilation

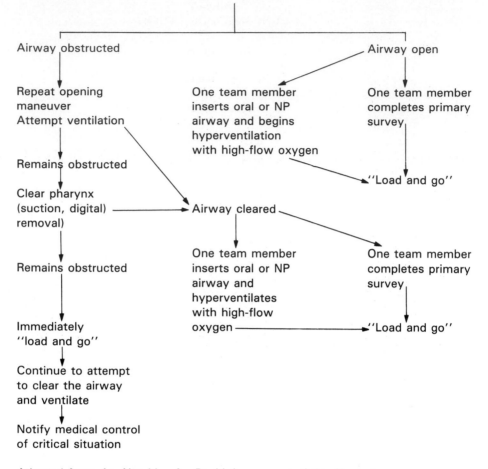

Adapted from *An Algorithm for Rapid Assessment of the Airway* by Daniel L. Cavallaro and Patricia J. Mominee

Chapter 5

CHEST TRAUMA

Anatomy

The thorax is a bony cage that encloses the following:

1. Heart
2. Lungs
3. Aorta
4. Superior and inferior vena cava
5. Trachea and bronchi
6. Esophagus
7. Diaphragm
8. Spinal cord

Also lying within the bounds of the rib cage are the

1. Kidneys
2. Spleen
3. Liver
4. Pancreas
5. Stomach

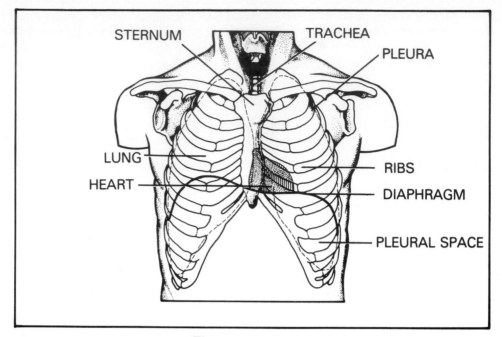

Figure 5–1. Thorax.

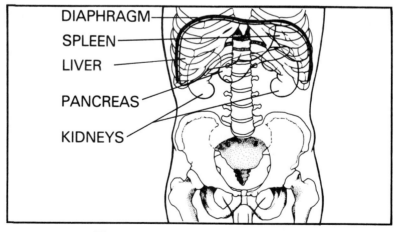

Figure 5–2. Intrathoracic abdomen.

Thus trauma to the body in the area covered by the rib cage can injure any one or several of the structures listed. Here again, you must be alert to the history of the injury and to the scene of the injury in order to be aware of mechanisms of injury. Then a careful, systematic evaluation, keeping in mind possible injuries, must be made.

EXAMPLE: A deceleration injury in which a car struck a tree and the driver hit the steering wheel should make you think immediately of the following:

1. Pneumothorax, hemothorax, or tension pneumothorax
2. Rib fractures
3. Sternal fracture
4. Myocardial contusion
5. Cardiac tamponade
6. Flail chest
7. Thoracic aorta tear
8. Spinal cord injury

You must keep priorities in mind as you evaluate the chest since several of the injuries require "load and go" treatment.

In this section we consider primarily injuries to the chest and structures above the diaphragm. Those structures in the intrathoracic abdomen are covered in Chapter 9.

Pathophysiology

Since there are so many systems involved, pathophysiology will be discussed with each specific injury. When you are evaluating a victim, always think of the most dangerous injuries first so as to give your patient the greatest chance of survival. If you do a great job splinting an ankle but your patient dies of an airway obstruction, you will never develop the reputation of a lifesaver.

I. **Injuries capable of producing death within a few moments**
    A. *Airway obstruction*
        1. Evaluation of the airway is always the first priority in evaluating any patient. You must look, listen, and feel for movement of air.
        2. If the victim is making respiratory effort but no air is moving or if he is making no respiratory effort, the airway must be opened immediately. Remember to stabilize the cervical spine while gaining control of the airway.
    B. *Open pneumothorax (sucking chest wound)*
        1. *Pathophysiology:* Normally, the chest expands and the diaphragm contracts, causing a negative pressure inside the chest. Air rushes in through the upper airway and trachea and expands the lungs. When the diaphragm and chest relax, a posi-

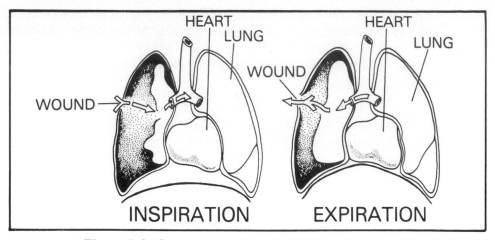

Figure 5–3. Open pneumothorax—sucking chest wound.

tive pressure is formed that forces the air back out the same route. If the chest sustains a penetrating injury (e.g., knife or missile) large enough to remain open, air will enter and exit the wound with the change of intrathoracic pressure; however, this air will only enter the pleural space (causing the lung to collapse). The air in the pleural space will not enter the lung and therefore will not contribute to oxygenation of the blood. Air will follow the path of least resistance, so if the opening is larger than the glottic opening, more air will enter the pleural space than the lungs. In other words, the movement of the ribs and diaphragm will be unable to form enough negative pressure to ventilate the lungs, and the victim will smother as surely as if he had an airway obstruction.

2. *Diagnosis of sucking chest wound:* There is generally no difficulty with this diagnosis. The patient will have sustained some sort of penetrating trauma to the chest, he will have trouble moving air even though his airway is open, and generally, he will have another opening in the chest that you can both see and hear.

3. *Treatment of sucking chest wound*
   a. Close the wound. This can be done with anything that will seal the wound. Have the patient exhale just before you seal the opening. A gel defibrillator pad (Littman, 3M) works best because it will stick to wet or dry skin. Petrolatum gauze or Saran wrap® also works well. You may

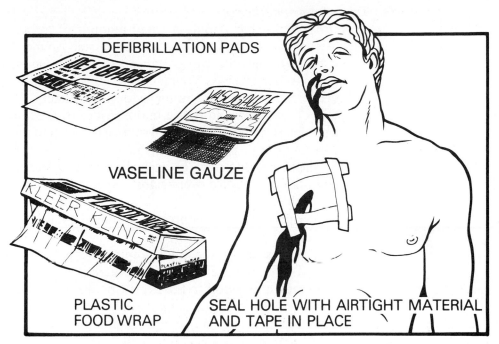

Figure 5-4. Treatment of sucking chest wound.

tape this dressing in place, but tape only three sides so there will be a route for air to escape if a tension pneumothorax begins to develop. A more sophisticated dressing can be made by cutting the tip out of a condom and taping the base of the condom over the opening. This will keep air from entering the chest but will allow air to exit, thus preventing any chance of a tension pneumothorax. For larger wounds, a thin rubber glove with the tip of a finger cut off can be used in the same manner. However, time is so important in this situation that the simpler procedure (defibrillator pad or Saran wrap®) is better.

b. Give oxygen.
c. If there is no danger of spinal injury (stab wound only), you may transport the victim on the affected side. This allows the uninjured lung to function best. If there is any danger of spinal injury, the victim must be transported supine on a spine board with neck stabilized.
d. Notify medical control so that they can have the surgeon and operating room available when you arrive.

C. *Tension pneumothorax*
  1. *Pathophysiology:* If only a small amount of air enters the chest, as usually happens with a bullet or stab wound, the lung on the affected side will collapse to a degree equal to the amount of air entering. Young people without preexisting lung disease can tolerate this injury with no difficulty. If the injury is more severe so that a major injury to the lung tissue or bronchus is present, air may continue to leak into the pleural space. As the air pressure in the pleural space rises, the lung on the affected side is collapsed and eventually the mediastinum is pushed over against the other lung. This causes two problems:
     a. The good lung is compressed so that ventilation is almost impossible.
     b. The pressure on the mediastinum collapses the superior and inferior vena cava so that there is marked decrease in return of blood to the heart (the distended neck veins seen in this condition are a sign of this collapse of the vena cava). Thus the victim becomes rapidly hypoxic from lack of ventilation and subsequently becomes shocky from

Figure 5–5. Pathophysiology of tension pneumothorax.

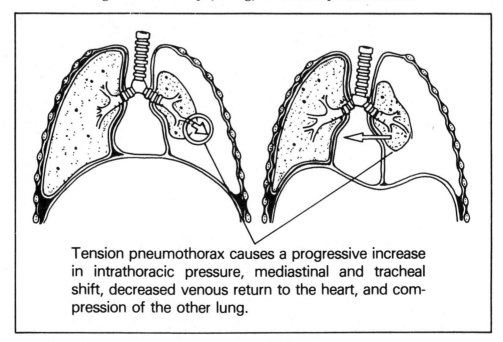

Tension pneumothorax causes a progressive increase in intrathoracic pressure, mediastinal and tracheal shift, decreased venous return to the heart, and compression of the other lung.

hypoxia and decreased cardiac output. Death occurs rapidly once the signs of shock appear.

2. *Diagnosis of tension pneumothorax*

   a. There will be a history of penetrating wound to the chest or a deceleration injury (motor vehicle accident or fall) that may have produced a tear of the bronchus or lung. Remember, a penetrating wound is not necessary to develop a tension pneumothorax.

   b. *Physical findings:* The patient will be in respiratory distress and will appear cyanotic (blue or dusky) and shocky.. He will move air poorly or not at all even with his airway open. Neck veins usually will be distended (unless hypovolemic), the trachea usually will be deviated away from the side of the injury. The trachea should be in the center of the sternal notch. The side of the chest in which the tension pneumothorax occurs will have absent or decreased breath sounds and will be hyperresonant to percussion because of air trapped in the chest.

3. *Treatment of tension pneumothorax:* This injury cannot be stabilized in the field. You must immediately notify your

Figure 5–6. Physical findings of tension pneumothorax.

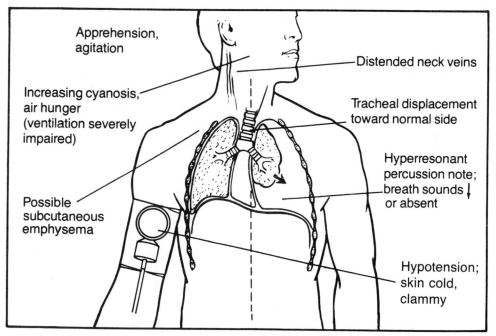

Apprehension, agitation

Increasing cyanosis, air hunger (ventilation severely impaired)

Possible subcutaneous emphysema

Distended neck veins

Tracheal displacement toward normal side

Hyperresonant percussion note; breath sounds ↓ or absent

Hypotension; skin cold, clammy

medical control physician and prepare to "load to go." This patient is dying of hypoxia, so give him oxygen at a wide-open rate. Assist ventilations as necessary. Transport without delay to the nearest staffed emergency department.

D. *Flail chest*

   1. *Pathophysiology:* The chest is made up of a series of 12 ribs, each of which connects to the sternum and vertebral column to form a circle. If a fracture occurs in one place in one or more ribs, the chest remains stable and the thorax can expand and contract normally. However, if two or more adjoining ribs are fractured in more than one place, the section becomes unstable and normal respiration cannot occur. This unstable section will respond to changes in chest pressure just as air does. When the rest of the chest expands, creating a negative intrathoracic pressure, the flail section will suck in. When the rest of the chest relaxes, creating positive pressure in the chest, the flail section will be pushed out. This motion of the flail segment is "paradoxical" or opposite to the rest of the chest wall. Great force is usually required to break multiple ribs in multiple places, so there is usually severe contusion to the underlying lung. There may also be associated pneumothorax,

Figure 5–7. Pathophysiology of flail chest.

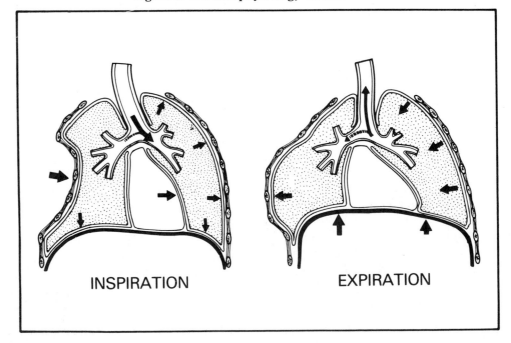

INSPIRATION   EXPIRATION

hemothorax, or both. Depending on the size of the flail seg-ment, there may be severe difficulty with ventilation. Air may actually be sucked back and forth between the two lungs rather than in and out through the trachea. This causes rapid hypoxia. Myocardial contusion is often associated with anterior flail chest.

2. *Diagnosis of flail chest:* There is always a history of chest trauma from a motor vehicle accident or fall. The victim will usually be moving air poorly in spite of an open airway. In-spection of the chest reveals an unstable section of thorax that moves in a paradoxical manner with respiration. Other injuries are often present and the patient may be in shock from associated injuries, hypoxia, or myocardial contusion.

3. *Treatment of flail chest*
   a. First stablize the flail segment with your hands to improve ventilation. Next, start oxygen and strap a sandbag or small cushion over the flail section to maintain stability of the chest wall. If the victim is in hemorrhagic shock from a hemothorax or other injuries, it is reasonable to use the antishock garment (MAST), but it might be pru-dent not to use the abdominal section. Blowing up the ab-

Figure 5–8. Physical findings of flail chest.

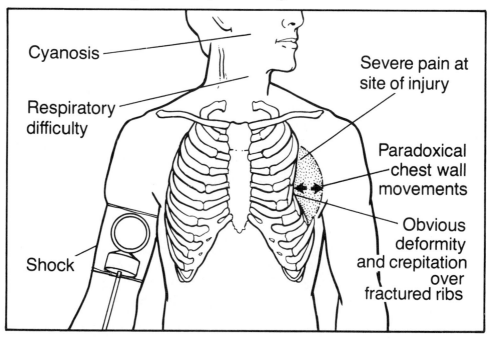

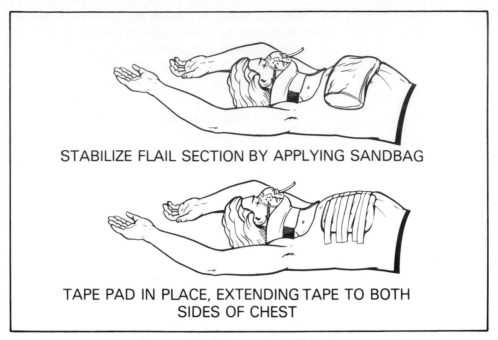

STABILIZE FLAIL SECTION BY APPLYING SANDBAG

TAPE PAD IN PLACE, EXTENDING TAPE TO BOTH
SIDES OF CHEST

Figure 5–9. Treatment of flail chest.

dominal section causes pressure on the diaphragm and decreases ventilation slightly. The victim has a real problem with ventilation and may not be able to tolerate any further decrease. You should transport without delay.

    b. In the past it has been suggested that victims with flail chest could be turned onto the affected side in order to stabilize the flail segment. This should never be done because there is always a possibility of spinal injury in this situation. All victims who have suffered a flail chest should be stabilized supine on a backboard.

The first four injuries had as their primary presenting symptom difficulty with respiration. The next three (hemothorax, myocardial contusion, and pericardial tamponade) are primarily circulatory problems.

E. *Massive hemothorax*

    1. *Pathophysiology:* Injuries to lung tissue usually do not cause excessive bleeding because circulation through the lung is under low pressure compared with the rest of the body, and lung tissue is rich in blood clotting factors, so injuries tend to seal themselves rapidly. Massive bleeding into the chest is usually

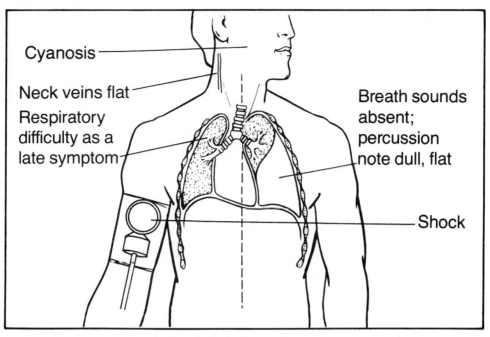

Cyanosis

Neck veins flat

Respiratory difficulty as a late symptom

Breath sounds absent; percussion note dull, flat

Shock

Figure 5–10. Physical findings of massive hemothorax.

caused by an injury to the heart or one of the major intra-thoracic blood vessels. Hemothorax may be associated with pneumothorax and may even, although rarely, be a tension hemopneumothorax.

2. *Diagnosis of massive hemothorax:* Hemothorax presents as shock primarily with ventilatory problems developing later. The patient will have dullness to percussion on the side of the hemothorax. Neck veins will be flat because the patient is hypovolemic.

3. *Treatment of massive hemothorax:* After initial evaluation, you should recognize this as a critical trauma situation. Rapid transport to an emergency facility capable of doing chest surgery is of utmost importance. You should notify medical control early so that arrangements can be made to have a thoracic surgeon available when you arrive. During transport, you must treat the underlying problem of hemothorax; hypovolemic shock. Treatment includes antishock garment, high-flow oxygen, and ventilatory assistance if needed. Massive hemothorax (especially from penetrating wounds to the chest) is the classic "load and go" situation.

Table 5–1 *Comparison of Tension Pneumothorax and Hemothorax*

	Tension pneumothorax	*Hemothorax*
Primary presenting symptom	Difficulty breathing, then shock	Shock, then difficulty breathing
Neck veins	Distended	Flat
Breath sounds	Decreased or absent on side of injury	Decreased or absent on side of injury
Percussion of chest	Hyperresonant	Dull
Tracheal deviation away from the side of the injury	Present	Usually not present

   F.   *Myocardial contusion*
      1.   *Pathophysiology:* The heart lies just behind the sternum and anterior ribs. Any blunt trauma to the anterior chest transmits force to the heart muscle. Bruising of the heart is essentially the same type of injury as a heart attack and shows up with the same symptoms: pain, dysrhythmias, and/or cardiogenic shock.
      2.   *Diagnosis of myocardial contusion:* You must have a high index of suspicion in any blunt trauma to the anterior chest. Approximately 10 percent of steering wheel injuries reportedly cause myocardial contusion. As stated above, the symptoms are the same as for a myocardial infarction or cardiac tamponade.
      3.   *Treatment of myocardial contusion:* Treatment is the same as for a heart attack victim. Give oxygen, watch for irregular heartbeat, and transport carefully. If the victim develops shock, you may try the antishock garment. If the shock is due to cardiac tamponade, the victim may improve. If the victim worsens or develops difficulty breathing, the shock is probably cardiogenic and the garment must be deflated.
   G.   *Cardiac tamponade*
      1.   *Pathophysiology:* The pericardium is a fibrous membrane that encloses the heart. Bleeding into the pericardium can be caused by penetrating injuries or blunt trauma to the heart. The pericardium will not stretch rapidly, so if blood collects between the pericardium and the heart, pressure will be applied to the heart muscle, squeezing it until the chambers of the heart are so small that not enough blood can be pumped to serve the body. As the pressure rises, neck veins distend. The

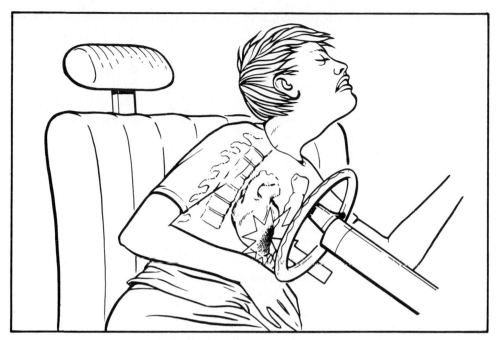

Figure 5–11. Pathophysiology of myocardial contusion.

Figure 5–12. Pathophysiology and physical findings of cardiac tamponade.

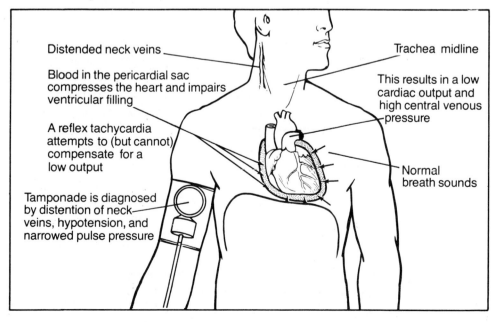

heart sounds become muffled because the heart is surrounded by a layer of blood and the pulse pressure narrows because the stroke volume is decreasing.

2. *Diagnosis of cardiac tamponade:* The patient will have a history of blunt or penetrating trauma to the chest. He will be in shock with distended neck veins, yet there will be bilateral breath sounds and the trachea will not be deviated. The pulse pressure will be decreased (but this occurs with all shock), and the heart sounds will be muffled (this occurs in most shock also). Essentially, you must suspect this injury in all patients with chest trauma and differentiate it from tension pneumo-thorax.

3. *Treatment of cardiac tamponade:* This is an injury that is rapidly fatal and cannot be treated in the field. This is a critical trauma situation, you must "load and go." You can give high-flow oxygen and apply the antishock garment, which may in-crease the venous pressure enough to increase cardiac filling and cardiac output. Remember that myocardial contusion with cardiogenic shock presents in the same way; if the victim worsens after application of the antishock garment, deflate it immediately.

H. *Impaled objects:* The most common are knives; however, other objects, from arrows to fence posts, have been encountered. The actual injury depends on what the object penetrates inside the chest. At the very least you have a sucking chest wound. You must not remove the impaled object, as it may have penetrated a large blood vessel; removing it might allow the victim to bleed to death immediately. Impaled objects are always removed by a surgeon in the operating room. The same holds true of impaled objects anywhere else in the body except the cheek of the face. There you can safely remove an impaled object since you can reach inside the mouth and put pressure on both sides of the wound to stop bleeding. For an object in the chest, the procedure is to stabilize the impaled object in place (yes, even a fence post), and seal around it if necessary to prevent a sucking chest wound. Petrolatum gauze works well for sealing. Transport rapidly to the emergency department while notifying medical control so that they can be prepared for the victim.

II. **Other chest injuries**
These are mentioned separately because either they are generally not fatal or they are not treatable in the field.

A. *Aortic disruption:* This is the most common cause of sudden death in an automobile accident or a fall from a height. The aorta tears in the arch, and the patient bleeds to death within a matter of seconds. Ninety percent of these patients die on the spot. Ten percent will have an incomplete tear that does not blow out until later, and they can be saved if the diagnosis is made in the emergency department. You cannot make this diagnosis in the field, but if your scene survey reveals severe deceleration forces, notify the emergency physician.

B. *Diaphragmatic hernias:* In deceleration injuries where blunt trauma to the abdomen (seat belt injury) occurs, the sudden increased intraabdominal pressure may tear the diaphragm and force the contents of the abdomen up into the chest. This usually presents with ventilatory symptoms much like pneumothorax and is treated with oxygen. Some victims may require respiratory assistance.

C. *Simple pneumothorax:* Most patients with normal lung function can tolerate even a complete pneumothorax on one side. Symptoms, if present, will be related to ventilation. Oxygen is generally all that is required until the patient reaches the hospital. You must continuously monitor the patient to be sure that a tension pneumothorax does not develop.

D. *Simple rib fractures:* This is the most common injury to the chest. It is usually caused by blunt trauma and generally presents as pain with respiration. A pneumothorax may frequently be associated with this injury. Be alert to the possible development of pneumothorax or hemothorax, and observe the patient to be sure that a flail segment is not present. Give oxygen if the victim is short of breath.

E. *Sternum fractures:* Blunt trauma to the anterior chest may break the sternum. You can usually diagnose this by palpation. Myocardial contusion and pericardial tamponade are often associated with fractures of the sternum.

Important Points to Remember

1. Remember the "ABCs."
2. Call medical control early; many of these patients require rapid transport to the emergency department. Your medical control physican will help you decide which patients you need to "load and go."

3. Immobilize the spine.
4. Penetrating wounds to the chest may produce shock by these means:
   a. Massive hemothorax
   b. Pericardial tamponade
   c. Tension pneumothorax
   d. Injury to the spine with spinal shock (remember to record your brief neurological examination)
5. Until proven otherwise, assume that trauma patients in shock with no external bleeding have internal bleeding. Also remember to check for tension pneumothorax and cardiac tamponade.

Chapter 6

SHOCK

Shock is a state of inadequate blood flow to the organs of the body. Not enough oxygen and nutrients are being delivered to the cells to keep them alive. Normal tissue perfusion requires four intact mechanisms:

A. Functioning pump: the heart

B. Adequate volume of fluid: the blood and plasma

C. Adequate air exchange to get oxygen into the blood

D. Intact vascular system to deliver blood to the tissue

The many clinical shock syndromes arise from the failure of one or more of these mechanisms.

A. *Failure of the pump*
  1. Cardiogenic shock
      a. Myocardial contusion
      b. Myocardial infarction (heart attack)
  2. Pericardial tamponade
B. *Lack of fluid volume*
  1. Blood loss (hemorrhagic shock)
  2. Fluid loss
      a. Burns
      b. Vomiting or diarrhea

C. *Lack of adequate air exchange*
   1. Airway obstruction
   2. Open pneumothorax
   3. Tension pneumothorax
   4. Flail chest
   5. Toxic gas inhalation
D. *Lack of adequate vascular system*
   1. Leaking vascular system: results in lack of fluid volume
   2. Dilated vascular system: results in too much space and relative lack of volume
      a. Spinal shock
      b. Anaphylactic shock
      c. Septic shock

Among trauma victims, shock is caused almost overwhelmingly from hypovolemic (blood loss) or lack of adequate air exchange. Spinal shock occurs much less commonly. Recognizing and treating shock in the early stages is one of the most important steps in increasing the survival rate of trauma victims. Since most basic EMTs are unable to use intravenous fluids or advanced airway interventions in the resuscitation of shock, they must be even more alert to the early signs of shock.

Hypovolemic shock is a clinical syndrome in which there is insufficient fluid (blood or plasma) to maintain pressure in the vascular system. Blood flow becomes so sluggish that the organs of the body die from lack of oxygen and nutrients. Hemorrhagic shock is a type of hypovolemic shock caused by an injury to the vascular system with resulting loss of enough blood to compromise tissue perfusion. Burn shock is also a type of hypovolemic shock in which plasma is lost instead of whole blood. With spinal shock there may be no actual loss of blood from the body. The blood simply pools in the large dilated vascular system and does not return to the heart. The effect is the same as if that pooled blood were lost. The circulation becomes too sluggish to maintain oxygen and food to the cells; therefore, the body organs die.

Pathophysiology of Hypovolemic Shock

As the blood volume decreases, the amount of blood returning to the heart decreases, which causes the amount of blood pumped to decrease. This all results in a decrease in the blood pressure. Receptors in the aorta and great vessels detect this decrease in pressure and signal the release of catecholamines (epinephrine and norepinephrine). Catecholamines cause:

1. Vasoconstriction in the less vital organs (skin and muscles) in order to raise the perfusion pressure in the vital organs
2. Increased rate and strength of contraction of the heart to raise the blood pressure
3. Sweating (not a useful response to shock but simply an effect of catecholamine release)

These effects combine to maintain the blood pressure and perfusion until the fluid loss can be replaced. If the loss continues, the perfusion pressure of the body will eventually become too low to maintain aerobic metabolism. At this point, since not enough oxygen is present, anaerobic metabolism begins. The by-products of anaerobic metabolism are large amounts of lactic and pyruvic acids. As the tissue becomes more and more acidotic, there is eventual loss of response to catecholamines. This results in vasodilation and sudden pooling of what little blood is left, causing precipitous loss of blood pressure and often ventricular fibrillation (acidotic, anoxic heart muscle) and death.

Symptoms of Hypovolemic Shock

The symptoms of hypovolemic shock reflect the basic physiologic mechanisms:

1. *Confusion, restlessness, or combativeness:* decreased blood flow to the brain
2. *Weakness:* hypoxia, acidosis
3. *Thirst:* low blood volume
4. *Pallor:* vasoconstriction secondary to effects of catecholamines
5. *Tachycardia (pulse > 100 per minute):* cardiac response to catecholamines
6. *Sweating (diaphoresis):* response of sweat glands to catecholamines
7. *Tachypnea (respiratory rate > 24 per minute):* hypoxia, acidosis
8. *Cold skin:* vasoconstriction of skin from catecholamines
9. *Hypotension (blood pressure < 100 systolic):* loss of blood volume

Classification of Hypovolemic Shock

Early shock: loss of approximately 15 to 25 percent of the blood volume (1.5 to 2.5 pints). This is associated with only slight to moderate tachycardia, pallor, narrowed pulse pressure, thirst, weakness, and delayed capillary refill. *Low blood pressure is not usually a symptom.*

Late shock: loss of approximately 30 to 45 percent of the blood volume (3 to 5 pints). This is associated with hypotension (low blood pressure) and *all* the other symptoms of hypovolemic shock listed above.

Test for Early Shock: Capillary Blanch Test

This is an early test for class II hemorrhage. Press on the victim's fingernail or the palm of his hand. The test is positive if the blanched area lasts longer than 2 seconds. This is an example of a test that means something if it is positive but means nothing if it is negative. If capillary refill is delayed, you have strong evidence of early shock. If capillary refill is normal, you do not have evidence that shock is not present.

Most trauma victims are young. Young people have very strong vasomotor responses to catecholamines. Falling blood pressure may be the last sign of shock in these victims. If you wait for them to have hypotension before treating their shock, you may be too late to save them. They often maintain a near-normal blood pressure until they are very acidotic, then have a sudden drop in blood pressure often associated with vomiting and aspiration and even cardiac arrest.

Pathophysiology of Inadequate Air Exchange

Airway obstruction physically prevents oxygen from entering the lungs, so no oxygenation of the blood occurs. Death follows in only a few minutes. Removing the obstruction immediately cures the shock, as long as irreversible damage has not occurred. Open pneumothorax collapses a lung as well as preventing adequate air exchange through the trachea. Sealing the opening provides immediate adequate temporary treatment. Tension pneumothorax both collapses the lungs and prevents return of blood to the heart. Decompression provides immediate relief. Inhalation of certain gases (smoke, carbon monoxide, etc.) causes inadequate air exchange because of displacement of oxygen from the lung, injury to the airways, or injury to the oxygen-carrying capacity of the blood. You must be aware that these victims will die within a very short time if their condition is not corrected. They will also almost all improve immediately with the correct treatment. Early recognition and transport is extremely important in this group.

Pathophysiology of Spinal Shock

The normal circulating adult blood volume is about 5 liters. The vascular system can hold many times this amount. A certain number of vessels are kept constricted at all times in order to maintain a normal blood pressure.

After a meal, blood is shunted to the intestines to absorb the food. During this time vessels in the muscles are constricted. If one attempts to exercise immediately after a meal, muscle cramps may develop because of poor blood flow in the muscles. Nausea and vomiting may also occur because of poor blood flow in the gastrointestinal tract. Control of vasoconstriction of the necessary vessels to maintain blood pressure is maintained through messages sent down the spinal cord from the higher centers. If the spinal cord is injured, no messages are sent to cause vasoconstriction, thus all the vessels remain open and the blood pools in the body and does not return to the heart. When the receptors in the aorta and great vessels detect a drop in blood pressure there is no way to send messages to the adrenal glands to secret epineprine (adrenalin) and norepinephrine. The pooling of the blood continues and blood pressure falls to shock levels. Eventually, acidosis from anaerobic metabolism causes cardiac arrest.

Symptoms of Spinal Shock

1. *Hypotension (blood pressure < 100 systolic):* loss of circulating blood volume.
2. *Confusion:* decreased perfusion of the brain. This is not as pronounced as would be expected. The victim is usually not restless or combative because he is paralyzed from his spinal injury.
3. *Weakness:* paralysis from spinal injury as well as hypoxia and acidosis.
4. *Tachypnea (respiration > 24 per minute):* Hypoxia and acidosis. This is usually diaphragmatic breathing only because the chest muscles are paralyzed.

The clinical presentation of spinal shock differs from hypovolemic shock in that there is no catecholamine release thus no pallor, tachycardia, or sweating. The victim will have a decreased blood pressure but the pulse will be slow, the skin warm, dry, and pink. The victim will often be more alert than would be expected for his blood pressure.

Important Points When Evaluating the Shock Victim

1. Young people often lose 30 percent of their blood volume before they get a drop in blood pressure. Do not base your diagnosis of shock on hypotension.
2. It is easy to underestimate the severity of blood loss until it is too late.
3. Hypotension, tachycardia, and pallor indicate bleeding into the chest or abdomen if no obvious external injuries are present.

4. Hypotension is almost never due to head injury; look elsewhere for blood loss.

5. The degree of head injury cannot be assessed accurately in the presence of deep shock.

6. The smell of alcohol should not influence your assessment in the emergency situation.

7. If the patient is confused, think of head injury or shock before attributing the confusion to alcohol intoxication.

8. Although there may be early shock and late shock, or mild shock and deep shock, all shock means one thing—this patient is near death! All shock requires aggressive treatment if the victim is to survive.

Management of Hypovolemic and Spinal Shock

Begin with the routine treatment priorities:

1. Open the airway and control the cervical spine.
2. Assess breathing and circulation.
3. Stop the bleeding.
4. Recognize critical situation (shock).
5. Transport immediately.
6. Treat shock in route.
7. Notify medical control.
8. Do secondary survey in route.

While you are going through your assessment, you should attempt to get a history of the injury to help establish possible mechanisms of injury. It is also important to know about prior medical history and medications when you get this information. Look for a Medic Alert tag.

Secure a good airway if the victim is unconscious. Remember to stabilize the cervical spine. Give oxygen to all victims in shock. This is a syndrome of insufficient tissue oxygenation. Give 6 liters/min for nasal cannula and 12 liters/min for face mask (preferably nonrebreathing mask).

Stop the bleeding. This is usually done with pressure dressings or direct pressure on the wound; consider air splints or antishock garment. Use a tourniquet as a last resort. If you use a tourniquet, note on the run report (and the patient) the time it is applied.

Apply an antishock garment to treat the shock, and keep the patient warm. It takes energy to maintain a normal temperature, and it takes oxygen for energy: The patient in shock has no oxygen to spare. Monitor vital signs and level of consciousness at least every 5 minutes.

Transport the patient as soon as possible; do not waste his golden hour.

The Antishock Garment*

Principle

No one has proven how antishock garments work, but the most likely mechanism is an increase in peripheral resistance by way of circumferential compression. The important thing is that they do work. They improve blood pressure and cerebral circulation in the hemorrhagic and spinal shock victim. They may also be used to tamponade bleeding and immobilize fractures of the pelvis and lower extremities.

Indications for Use in Trauma

1. Systolic blood pressure less than 80 mmHg
2. Shocklike symptoms and systolic blood pressure of 100 mmHg or less
3. Pelvic fracture
4. Fracture of lower extremity
5. Spinal shock
6. Massive abdominal bleeding

Contraindications

1. Pulmonary edema
2. Abdominal injury with protruding viscera (may use leg compartments)
3. Pregnancy (may use leg compartments)

Head injuries do not produce shock. If a patient with a head injury develops symptoms of shock, he probably has hypovolemic shock from internal or external blood loss, or he may have spinal shock. This is not a contraindication to the use of the antishock garment. The use of the antishock garment improves cerebral circulation, decreases cerebral ischemia, and inhibits the development of cerebral edema.

Thoracic injuries also are not a contraindication to the use of MAST. In a situation in which thoracic injuries exist, you should try to raise the systolic blood pressure only to the range 100 to 110 mmHg.

*Also known as military antishock trousers or MAST.

Use of the Antishock Garment

The technique of applying and removing the garment is covered in Skill Station 5. Three variations of the garment are available:

1. Plain garment with no pressure gauges
2. Garment with one gauge that can be rotated among the three compartments
3. Garment with three gauges, one for each compartment

For trauma use the plain garment. It is superior since the only gauge you need is a blood pressure cuff on the patient's arm. The danger with having extra gauges is that one tends to become more concerned with the pressure in the suit than the pressure in the patient.

Important Points in the Use of the Antishock Garment

1. Application of the garment takes 1 to 2 minutes and immediately improves the patient's condition. Note the time of inflation on the run report.

Figure 6–1. Military anti-shock trousers (MAST)—no pressure gauges.

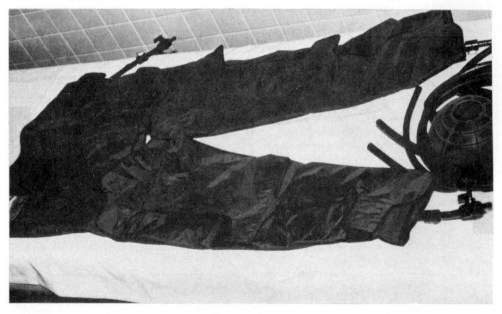

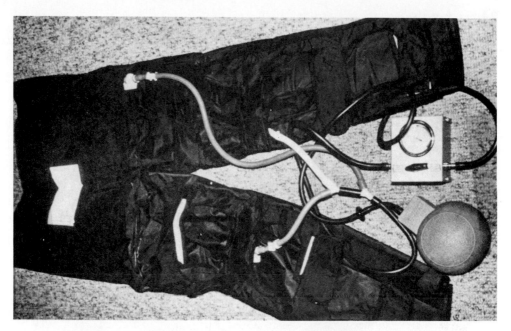

Figure 6–2. Military anti-shock trousers (MAST)—one pressure gauge.

Figure 6–3. Military anti-shock trousers (MAST)—three pressure gauges.

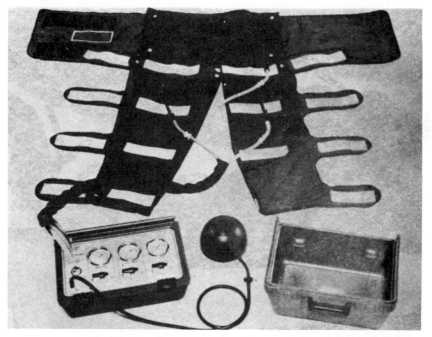

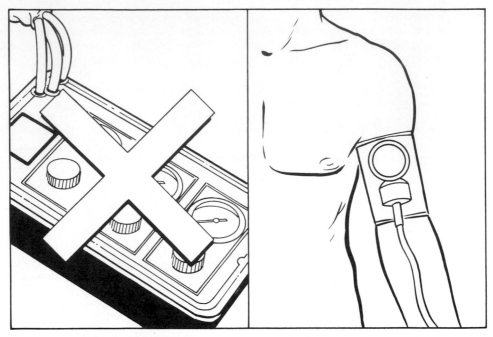

Figure 6–4. Blood pressure gauge and air pressure gauge for MAST. The pressure in the victim is what is important!

2. Transportation of a patient with the garment inflated will minimize displacement of pelvic and other fractures. If a traction splint is required, apply it after the garment is in place and then inflate the garment.

3. Once the garment has been placed on a patient, it should be removed in a hospital only under a physician's direction unless pulmonary edema develops. During removal there must be constant monitoring of the vital signs. A blood pressure drop of 5 mmHg signals a halt to deflation until more fluid can be replaced. The greatest danger associated with utilization of the suit is rapid removal by persons unaccustomed to its use.

Summary

Hemorrhagic shock is a critical condition that occurs just before death. In the past, treatment has tended to be "too little and too late." However, successful resuscitation is almost always possible if careful, alert evaluation is teamed with application of the antishock garment and early transport before the victim is in late shock.

Chapter 7

SPINAL CORD TRAUMA

Injuries to the spinal cord occur in over 10 percent of all multiple trauma patients and in 15 to 20 percent of all serious head injury patients. The most common victim of a spinal cord injury is an 18- to 35-year-old male who has been in an automobile accident. The initial evaluation and stabilization of the spinal cord injury victim will often determine whether that patient regains normal function or is crippled for life; in no other system evaluation is the rule "first do no harm" more important. Along with the physical and emotional trauma, there are other concerns as well. Today, the estimated cost of lifetime care for a paraplegic is about $1.5 million.

The key to preventing further spinal injury is thinking about the possibility of a spinal injury before the patient is moved. You must always look for possible mechanisms of spinal injuries. When in doubt, stabilize the spine: The patient will not be harmed by being transported on a spine board with the cervical spine immobilized. As a general rule, *all* trauma victims are considered to have a spinal injury until proven otherwise. Since you cannot rule out spinal injury in the field, all trauma victims are transported on a spine board with the neck stabilized.

Anatomy of the Spinal Column

The spinal column serves as the main axis of the body. It is flexible to some degree but provides rigidity to the trunk and neck. It is made up of 26 bones (vertebrae) that are divided into five segments:

1. *Cervical spine:* made up of the seven bones in the neck
2. *Thoracic spine:* made up of the 12 bones in the upper back to which the 12 ribs are attached
3. *Lumbar spine:* made up of the five bones in the lower back
4. *Sacrum:* part of the pelvic girdle
5. *Coccyx:* the tail bone

Each vertebra consists of a solid body and a vertebral arch through which passes the spinal cord and spinal nerve roots. Thus the spinal column also serves as a protector of the spinal cord. Each vertebra is separated by an intervertebral disc that serves as a cushion and allows motion in the spine.

Figure 7–1. Anatomy of spinal column.

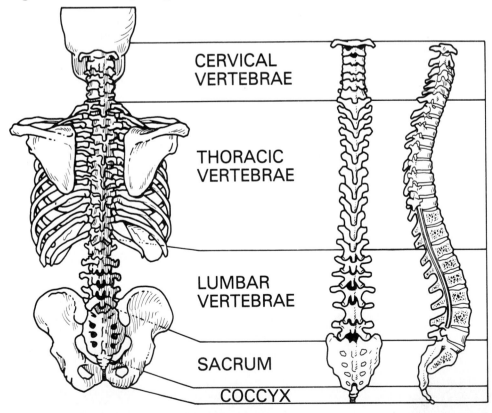

CERVICAL VERTEBRAE

THORACIC VERTEBRAE

LUMBAR VERTEBRAE

SACRUM

COCCYX

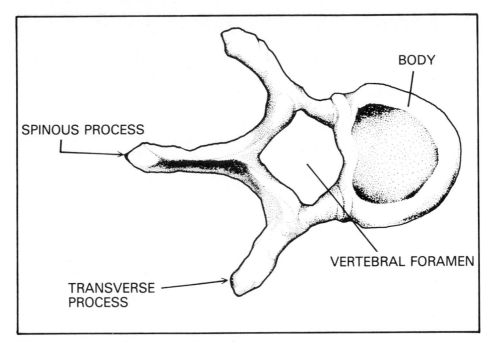

Figure 7–2. Vertebra viewed from above.

The Spinal Cord

The spinal cord is a continuation of the central nervous system outside the skull. It is like an electrical cable extending down through the vertebral foramen of the spinal column with nerve roots exiting between every pair of vertebrae. This is a two-way conduction system bringing sensory messages to the brain and sending motor messages to the muscles and organs. If the cord is transected at any point, there is complete loss of motor, sensory, and reflex activity below that area. Thus an injury to the lumbar area of the cord could cause paralysis of both legs but would not affect the arms. An injury in the neck could cause paralysis of both arms and both legs.

Fractures or dislocations of the spinal column may occur without injury to the spinal cord, but the potential for injury is always present and may become a reality with improper handling. Conversely, injury to the spinal cord may occur without fracture or dislocation of the vertebrae. Most injuries to the spine and spinal cord occur in the cervical spine because it is relatively unprotected compared with the rest of the spine. It is also poorly supported in most automobile seats. Since it is the stalk on which the head sits, any forces acting on the head are transmitted to the neck. The magnitude of these forces

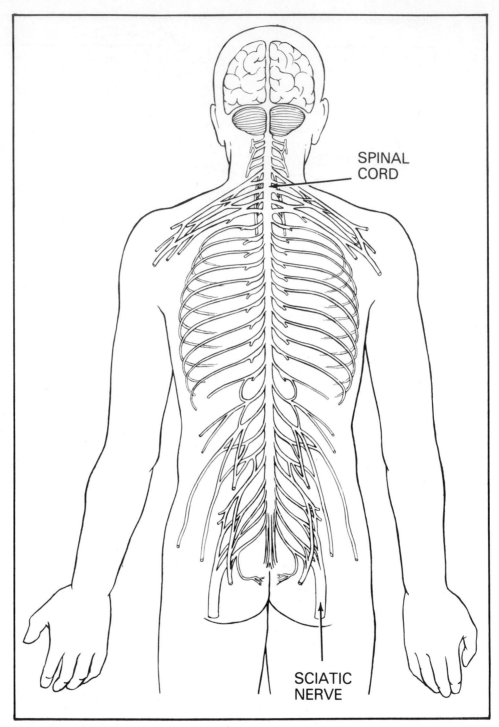

SPINAL CORD

SCIATIC NERVE

Figure 7–3. Spinal cord. The spinal cord is a continuation of the central nervous system outside of the skull.

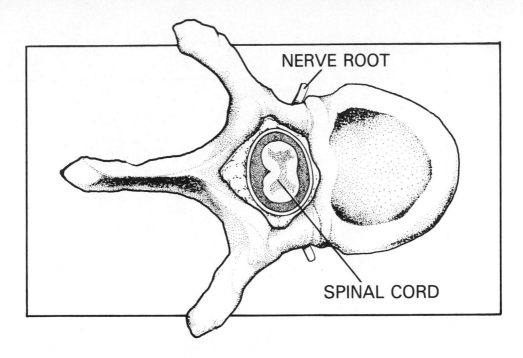

Figure 7–4. Relationship of spinal cord to vertebra.

is often very great and frequently causes fracture and dislocation of the cervical vertebrae, which, in turn, injures the spinal cord that passes through the small intervertebral foramen.

The thoracic spine is well stabilized by the rib cage and is usually well supported in most automobile seats. Thus it is injured much less often. If an injury does occur to the thoracic spine, there is high probability of spinal cord injury because the intervertebral foramen is smallest in this region of the spine.

If there is any possibility of injury to the spine, treat the patient as if an injury were present.

Causes of Spinal Injury

There are certain situations that should make you think immediately of the danger of spinal injury.

Motor Vehicle Accident

Any sudden deceleration injury can cause flexion or extension injury to the spine. This can happen even when seat belts are worn. All victims of motor vehicle accidents should be assumed to have spinal injuries until proven otherwise.

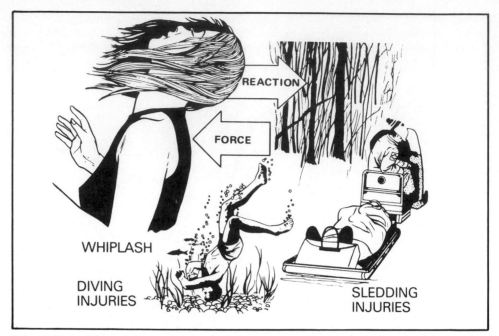

Figure 7–5. Mechanisms of injury.

Fall

The height of the fall and the manner in which the body strikes the ground determines where and what type of spinal injury may occur. Remember that there is the possibility of thoracic aortic injury here also. Falls in which the person lands on their feet are often associated with compression fractures of the lumbar spine. This is especially true if there is a fracture of the foot or ankle.

Diving

This tends to be a flexion injury to the cervical spine. It often occurs in the upper cervical spine and is a frequent cause of drowning. You must think of this injury if you are called to rescue a drowning victim. The victim's neck must be stabilized immediately while still in the water if there is a history of diving preceding the rescue.

Athletic Competition

High-risk sports include tackle football, surfing, wrestling, gymnastics, and trampoline. Cervical spine fractures are the number one cause of fatal football injuries.

Penetrating Trauma

Gunshot wounds to the neck, chest, or abdomen may directly penetrate the spinal cord. Knife wounds of the neck or back may penetrate or lacerate the cord.

Electric Shock

Spinal injury may occur from direct electrical injury or by the violent muscle spasm that accompanies electrical shock.

Sudden Twist

Often this is all it takes to cause herniation of a degenerated intervertebral disc into the intervertebral foramen, causing pressure on the spinal cord. You must consider this when there is a history of sudden, severe neck or back pain.

Specific Injuries

The spinal cord may be bruised, compressed, lacerated, or completely transected. The cord does not tolerate compression well—even for short periods.

Figure 7-6. Herniated intervertebral disc.

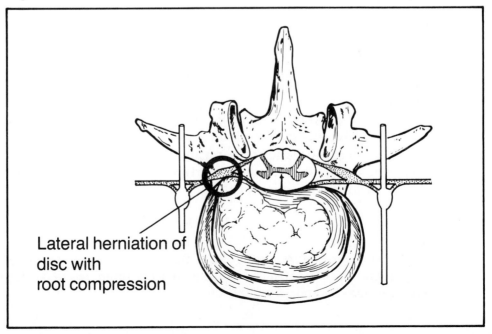

Lateral herniation of disc with root compression

There are two mechanisms of respiration: diaphragmatic breathing and breathing by expansion of the chest wall. Expansion of the chest wall is accomplished by contraction of the muscle between the ribs and is controlled by nerves coming out of the thoracic spinal cord at the same level. Injury to the cervical spine at any level will cause paralysis of this type of respiration. Diaphragmatic breathing is controlled by the phrenic nerve, which originates in the neck at the level of the third, fourth, and fifth cervical vertebrae. Spinal cord injuries above this level cause paralysis of both methods of respiration. Most of these victims will be dead at the scene unless you are there to ventilate them. Spinal cord injuries below the fifth cervical vertebrae cause paralysis of the chest wall but the diaphragm is still functional, thus the victim can still breathe. Victims who are paralyzed below the neck but still have diaphragmatic breathing (stomach rises when they breathe, but chest does not) have lower cervical spinal cord injury. A total disruption of the cord causes loss of motor function, sensation, and reflexes below the level of the injury. There can be various degrees of injury to the cord so that one or more functions may be lost but the others remain; thus you should quickly evaluate motor function and sensation in both hands and both feet.

Whiplash: Cervical Strain

This is the most common injury from a rear-end automobile collision. It is a hyperextension injury with tearing and stretching of the anterior neck muscles. A 15-mile-per-hour rear-end collision can accelerate the head backward with a force of 10 times the pull of gravity.

Spinal Shock: Neurogenic Shock

Spinal shock is caused by loss of the sympathetic control of the capillary bed. Thus there is such a large pooling of blood in the capillary bed that the blood pressure drops. Since there is no release of catecholamines (epinephrine and norepinephrine), there is no pallor or tachycardia. The patient with spinal shock will have a decreased blood pressure, but the pulse will be slow and strong, the skin will usually be warm and dry, and the patient may be oriented and alert. Spinal shock responds poorly to fluid replacement but is easily corrected with the application of the antishock garment.

Hypothermia

With spinal cord injury there is loss of thermoregulatory mechanisms, so if the patient is not covered, he can experience a rapid loss of body heat with resultant hypothermia.

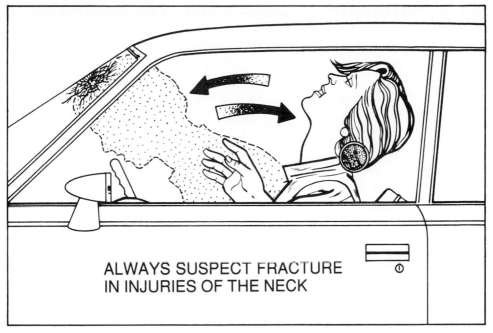

Figure 7–7. Cervical strain. Severe strain is usually evident from the history of the accident. Hyperextension or hyerflexion is often the mechanism of injury, which may involve either stretching or tearing of ligaments. Symptoms include neck immobility (caused by pain) and spasm of injured muscles.

Central Cord Syndrome

As mentioned before, injury to the spinal cord usually affects everything distal to that area. An injury to the cord in the neck causes weakness or paralysis in the arms, trunk, and legs. However, there is a particular situation in which this is not true. If there is bruising of the center of the spinal cord in the neck, the position of the motor and sensory nerves (arms are more medial—see illustration) will cause weakness or paralysis of the arms without the legs being affected.

Brief Neurological Examination for Possible Spinal Cord Injury

The purpose of this examination is to document loss of sensation and/or motor function. This does not have to be a detailed examination in the field. Parts of the examination obviously cannot be done in the unconscious patient.

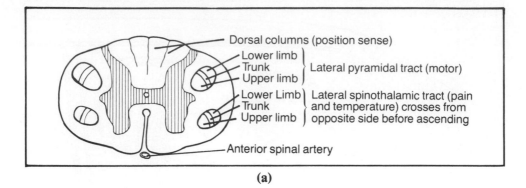

(a)

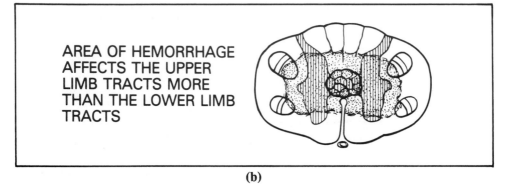

AREA OF HEMORRHAGE AFFECTS THE UPPER LIMB TRACTS MORE THAN THE LOWER LIMB TRACTS

(b)

Figure 7–8a. Spinal cord orientation.

Figure 7–8b. Central cord syndrome. Involves hemorrhage and edema of central cord. On either side of the cord, parts of the three main tracts are involved so that upper limbs are affected more than lower limbs.

1. *Sensory—conscious patient:* Ask if he can feel you touch him lightly on each hand and each foot. If he cannot feel light touch, try a pin-prick. If there is a sensory loss, record the level at which sensation stops; make a mark on the skin of the abdomen or chest with a ball-point pen.

2. *Motor—conscious or unconscious patient:* Ask him to move the fingers of each hand and toes of each foot. If the patient is unconscious, does he make any spontaneous movement? Does he move in response to pain?

3. *Reflexes:* This is probably not a useful examination in the field. A total transection of the cord will cause loss of sensation, motor function, and reflexes. If any sensation or motor function remains, there is a chance for recovery.

Priority Plan

Arrival at the Scene

You must make a quick assessment of the overall situation. Quickly note from the scene the apparent mechanisms of injury. All victims of motor vehicle accidents should be assumed to have spinal injury until proven otherwise. All unconscious patients as well as all head or facial injury victims should be assumed to have spinal injuries. Think of spinal injuries in falls, diving accidents, near drownings, gunshot wounds (of neck, chest, or abdomen), explosions, and electrocution injuries.

Initial Assessment of the Patient with Possible Spinal Injury

This begins immediately—even before extrication. Begin with routine assessment and treatment priorities.

1. Evaluate airway while controlling the spine. Check the initial level of consciousness. Have your partner immobilize the spine as you evaluate and secure the airway. Have him stabilize the head in a neutral position with his hands on either side of the head. Remember that the neck must not be extended when there is a chance of spinal cord injury. If the victim is face down, one rescuer must immobilize the neck in a neutral position while other rescuers log-roll the victim onto a spine board.

Figure 7–9. Modified jaw thrust.

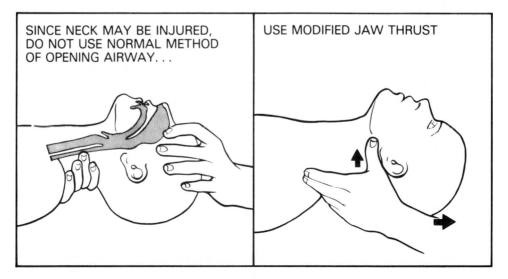

SINCE NECK MAY BE INJURED, DO NOT USE NORMAL METHOD OF OPENING AIRWAY...

USE MODIFIED JAW THRUST

2. Check breathing.
   a. As you check the breathing, you should also look at the neck (for neck vein distension, tracheal injury or deviation, and tenderness or abnormality of the cervical spine) and then apply a rigid extrication collar (foam-rubber choke collars are not adequate).
   b. Control circulation. If cardiopulmonary resuscitation is required, you must rapidly extricate the victim and place him on a firm surface. A spine board is perfect and also protects the thoracic and lumbar spine. Do not forget that drowning victims requiring cardiopulmonary resuscitation often have neck injuries (diving injury); if you extend the neck, you can cause complete paralysis. Always stabilize the neck while in the water if there is any possibility that a diving injury has occurred.
3. Stop significant bleeding.
4. Make decision about critical trauma situations. If critical situation is present, transfer to a long backboard and transport immediately. If critical situation is not apparent, transfer to a long backboard and begin secondary survey.
5. Perform secondary survey. As you do the secondary survey, have another EMT splint the fractures. Do your neurological examination now. Include level of consciousness, eye opening, pupils, ability to speak, bilateral movement of fingers and toes, and bilateral sensory examination. If there is a loss of sensation, record and mark the level on the patient.
6. Obtain a history of the injury:
   a. Personal observation
   b. Bystanders' observations
   c. Patient's description
   d. *Important points:* Was the patient moved before you arrived? For the paralyzed patient, did he have any movement before you arrived? Were there any changes in his condition before you arrived?
7. Document findings.
8. Transport with continuous monitoring.

Tips on Management

1. If there is an obvious spinal injury with paralysis, be sure to put the antishock garment on the spine board since the patient may go into spinal shock.
2. Be sure the patient is securely immobilized on the spine board. A patient with spinal injury is likely to vomit, so he and the board must be rolled to the side to prevent aspiration of vomitus.

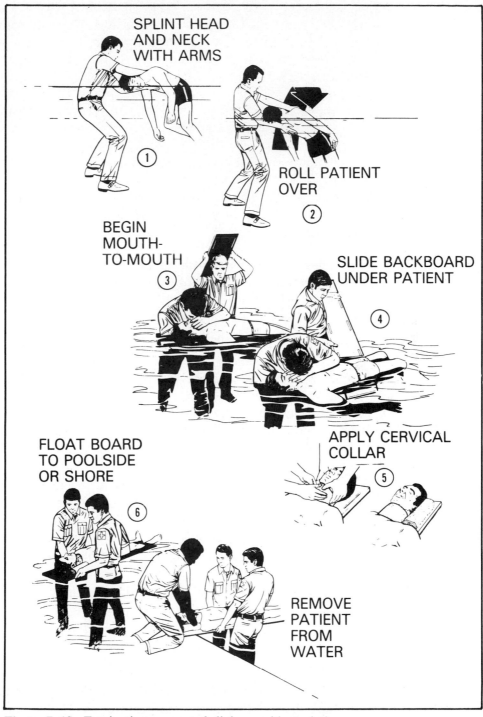

Figure 7–10. Extricating suspected diving accident victim.

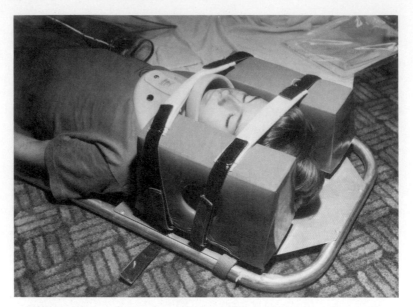

Figure 7–11. Spine board with rigid extrication collar and padded immobilization device. Collars do not give adequate lateral support—use padded immobilization device also.

3. Sandbags have been used for head immobilization and perform well when the victim is supine. However, if the board is tilted or the victim and board are rotated (as to prevent aspiration when patient vomits), the weight of the sandbags may cause a large degree of head movement. Lighter-weight bulky objects such as towel rolls, blanket rolls, or head cushions are a better tool for this job. When applied properly, these devices allow removal of the collar, which allows observation of the neck.

4. It is usually best to remove crash helmets in the field. You cannot manage the airway with some helmets (full face) still in place. Also, if the helmet is left in place, it may eventually be removed by someone not trained in the proper removal technique. If there is a neck injury, an improper technique during removal of the helmet could cause spinal injury (see Skill Station 6).

5. Do not allow the patient with possible spine injuries to sit or stand.

6. Cover the patient to prevent hypothermia.

Summary

Always be alert to mechanisms that may produce injuries of the spine. When in doubt, immobilze; your first duty is to prevent injury.

Chapter 8

HEAD TRAUMA

About 40 percent of trauma victims have central nervous system injuries. This group has a death rate twice as high as that of victims with other types of injuries (35 percent versus 17 percent overall). As with other injuries, rapid organized evaluation and treatments gives the patient the greatest chance for complete recovery. To understand evaluation and management of head injuries, you must have some knowledge of the basic anatomy and physiology of this area.

Anatomy of the Head

The head (excluding the face and facial structures) is made up of the following:

1. Scalp
2. Skull
3. Fibrous coverings of the brain
4. Brain substance
5. Cerebrospinal fluid
6. Vascular compartments

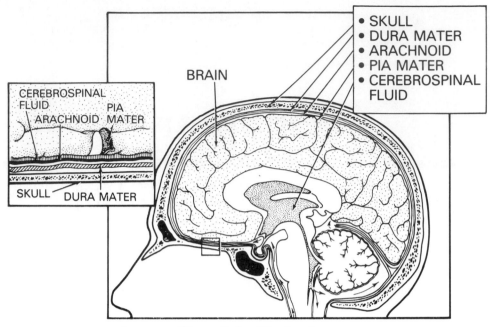

Figure 8–1.   The head.

The skull is like a closed box; the only significant opening is the foramen magnum at the base of the skull where the spinal cord exits. The rigid, unyielding nature of the skull is the basis of several injury mechanisms in head trauma.

Pathophysiology of Head Trauma

It is best to think of the brain as being fluid in nature. Most brain injuries are not from direct injury to brain tissue but occur due to the movement of the brain inside the skull. In deceleration injuries the head usually strikes some object, such as the windshield, which causes a sudden stop of the head and skull. Inside the skull, the brain moves forward like a wave, impacting first against the original blow and then rebounding and hitting the opposite side of the inner surface of the skull. Injuries may ocur to the brain in the area of the original blow (coup) or on the opposite side (contrecoup). This movement inside the skull causes most of the injuries seen after trauma.

The base of the skull is rough. Movement over this area causes various degrees of injury to the brain substance or blood vessels serving the brain.

The initial response of the bruised brain is swelling. This is from increased blood volume because of vasodilatation and increased cerebral blood flow to the injured areas. The buildup of this extra blood volume exerts pressure

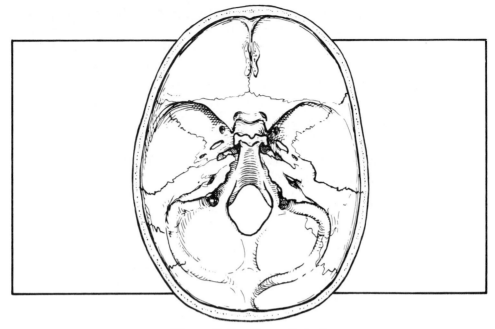

Figure 8-2.   Base of skull.

on the brain, eventually causing decreased blood flow to the uninjured parts of the brain. The buildup of increased cerebral water (edema fluid) does not occur immediately but develops over the next 24 to 48 hours. This is an important concept in that early efforts to decrease the vasodilatation in the injured areas can have a profound effect on the patient's eventual outcome.

The blood level of carbon dioxide (CO_2) has a critical effect on cerebral vessels. The normal blood level of carbon dioxide is 40 mmHg. Breathing faster lowers the CO_2 blood level, while slower breathing increases the blood level. Lowering the level of carbon dioxide (hyperventilation—rapid breathing) will cause the cerebral vessels to constrict and help prevent the accumulation of blood in the injured area. This prevents increased pressure on the brain. Conversely, if respiration slows down (the usual response to head injury), there will be vasodilatation and worsening of the pressure on the brain. If you immediately hyperventilate (>24 breaths per minute) the head injury victim, you can decrease the CO_2 level from 40 mmHg down to about 26 mmHg. This causes an immediate constriction of the cerebral vessels. This will help prevent the buildup of blood in the injured areas and allow better blood flow to the rest of the brain. Hyperventilation is a critical point in treatment of head injury. Early in the course of the injury, hyperventilation is more important than the administration of medication. Any victim who has decreased level of consciousness should have immediate hyperventilation.

Head injuries may be the result of bruising of the brain substance with resulting swelling and pressure on the rest of the brain, tearing of blood vessels with resulting bleeding and development of pressure on the brain, or direct penetrating injuries to the brain substance from foreign objects (e.g., bullets or knives) or pieces of bone from a skull fracture.

Intracranial Pressure

Inside the skull and fibrous coverings of the brain are the brain tissue, cerebrospinal fluid, and blood. Any increase in the size of one of these must be at the expense of the other two because the skull will not expand. The only part of the system that can "give" is the cerebrospinal fluid, but even if this fluid were completely "squeezed" out of the skull, there would be little extra space. Blood supply cannot be compromised, for the brain tissue must have a good continuous supply of blood to function. Since none of the components of the brain can be compromised, any swelling of the brain will cause an increase in intracranial pressure.

The pressure of the blood flowing through the brain is called the cerebral perfusion pressure. Cerebral perfusion pressure equals blood pressure minus intracerebral pressure (CPP = BP − ICP). Any increase in pressure inside the skull causes a decrease in the flow of blood to the brain. If the brain swells or if there is bleeding inside the skull, the intracerebral pressure increases and the perfusion pressure decreases. The body has a protective reflex (Cushing reflex) that works to maintain a constant flow of blood to the brain: If the intracerebral pressure increases, there will be a concurrent rise in blood pressure to try to maintain blood flow in the brain. This will continue until a critical point at which everything collapses and the victim dies. A very important point

Figure 8–3.   Cushing response.

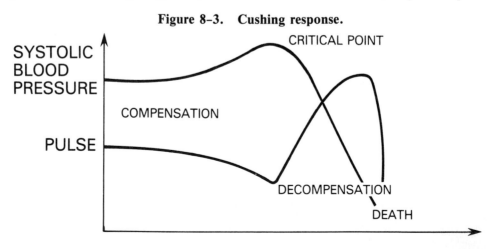

to remember here is that head injuries (if there is increased intracranial pressure) tend to cause an *increase* in blood pressure, so the presence of low blood pressure in a head injury patient is probably due to bleeding or spinal cord injury. Head injuries almost never are the cause of the shock. You must look for and treat the cause. Unexplained rises in blood pressure in a head trauma patient may indicate a worsening intracranial injury, causing increased intracranial pressure. Falling blood pressure from head trauma occurs only as a terminal event.

Anoxic Brain Injury

Injuries to the brain from lack of oxygen (e.g., cardiac arrest, choking, drowning) affect the brain differently from direct trauma. If the brain goes more than 4 to 6 minutes without oxygen, spasm develops in the small arteries so that if the brain is reperfused, blood will not flow to the cortex, and the patient will die within a day or so from brain failure. This arterial spasm is related to flow of calcium into the arterial muscle cells; complete spasm does not occur for approximately 90 minutes.

It has been long thought that except for cold water drownings, the brain could not be resuscitated after 4 to 6 minutes of anoxia. Exciting research into brain resuscitation gives hope of someday being able to save many victims that are presently unsalvageable.

Head Injuries

Scalp Wounds

The scalp is very vascular and can bleed extensively when cut. This can be very important in children who bleed as freely as adults but have much less blood volume to lose. As a general rule, adults with scalp injuries and shock usually have their shock caused by some other site of bleeding (often internal). Most bleeding from the scalp is easily controlled with direct pressure.

Skull Injuries

Skull injuries can be linear nondisplaced fractures, depressed skull fractures, and compound skull fractures. There is very little you can do in the field for these except to remember not to put pressure on an obvious depressed skull fracture. Penetrating objects in the skull should be stabilized in place and the victim transported immediately to the emergency room.

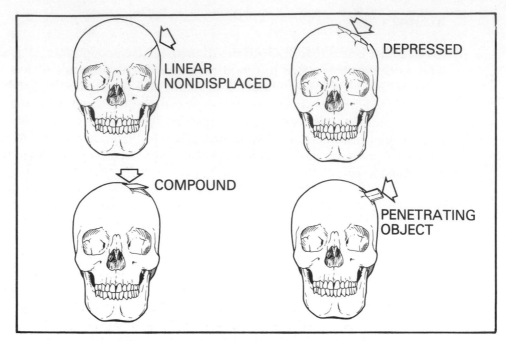

Figure 8–4.   Skull fracture—linear nondisplaced, depressed, compound, and penetrating object.

Brain Injuries

There are several types of brain injuries. The following outline briefly discusses some of these.

I.   Concussion

A concussion implies no significant injury to the brain itself. There is usually a history of trauma to the head with a variable period of unconsciousness or confusion and then a return to normal consciousness. There may be amnesia from the injury. This amnesia usually extends to some point before the injury so that often the patient will not remember the events leading to the injury. There may be dizziness, headache or nausea. This patient requires a period of observation; if unconsciousness lasts for 5 minutes or more, usually he should be admitted to the hospital for observation.

II.   Cerebral contusion

A cerebral contusion is a bruise of the brain. A patient with a cerebral contusion will have a history of prolonged unconsciousness or a serious change in his state of consciousness (e.g., will often ask the same question over and over). He may have focal neurological signs. This patient should be admitted for observation.

III. Intracranial hemorrhage

Bleeding can occur between the skull and the dura (the fibrous covering of the brain), between the dura and the brain, or in the brain tissue itself.

A. *Acute epidural hematoma:* This is a rare injury (less than 1 percent of head injuries) that is usually caused by a tear in the middle meningeal artery. It is often associated with a linear skull fracture in the temporal or parietal region. Because it is arterial bleeding, pressure can rise rapidly, so death may occur quickly. Surgical removal of the blood and ligation of the artery often gives excellent recovery, for often the underlying brain tissue is not injured. The symptoms include a history of head trauma with initial loss of consciousness followed by a period during which the patient is conscious and coherent. Later the patient will lapse into unconsciousness and develop a paralysis on the opposite side from the injury. There is usually a dilated and fixed pupil on the same side as the injury. Death usually follows rapidly. Since the early symptoms are the same as for concussion, this points out the importance of observation for victims who have ''only a concussion.'' The classic example of epidural hematoma is the boxer

Figure 8–5.   Acute epidural hematoma. This hemorrhage may follow injury to the extradural arteries. The blood collects between the fibrous dura and the periosteum.

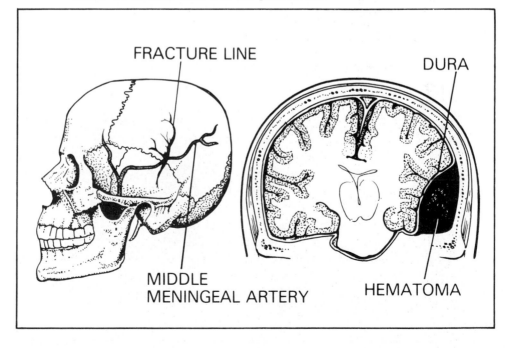

who is knocked unconscious, wakes up, and is allowed to go home, only to be found dead in bed the next morning.

B. *Acute subdural hematoma:* This is caused by bleeding between the dura and the brain substance. This injury is usually associated with injury to the underlying brain tissue. Because the bleeding is venous, pressure develops more slowly, and often the diagnosis is not made for hours after the injury. The signs and symptoms include headache, fluctuations in the level of consciousness, and eventually paralysis on the side opposite the injury. Because of injury to the brain tissue, the prognosis is often poor in spite of surgery. Mortality is very high (60 to 90 percent) in victims who are comatose when found. Recent studies have found that early surgery reduces mortality. The death rate for those patients on whom surgery is performed less than 4 hours following the injury is 30 percent. The death rate for surgery performed more than 4 hours after injury is 90 percent.

C. *Intracerebral hemorrhage:* This is bleeding within the brain tissue. It is always associated with penetrating injuries and may be associated with blunt trauma. Surgery is usually not helpful. Symptoms depend on the amount of injury and the areas involved.

Figure 8–6. Acute subdural hematoma. This usually occurs following the rupture of dural vessels (veins). Blood collects and often severely compresses and distorts the brain.

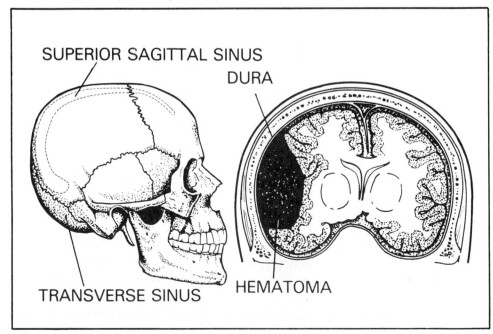

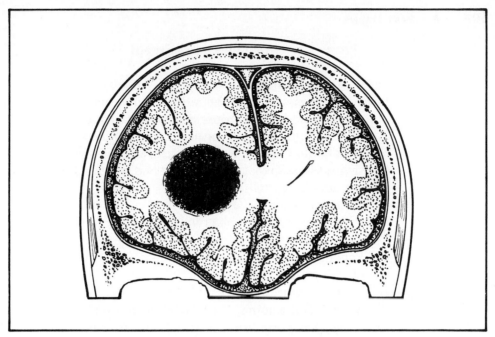

Figure 8-7. Intracerebral hemorrhage.

Evaluation of the Head Trauma Victim

Remember that every trauma victim is initially evaluated in the same sequence.

1. Secure airway, control the cervical spine, and note level of consciousness.
2. Assess breathing and circulation. Begin hyperventilation (>24 breaths per minute) of patients with decreased LOC.
3. Stop the bleeding.
4. Make decision about critical trauma situations. If a critical situation is identified, transfer to a long backboard and transport immediately. If a critical situation is not apparent, transfer the victim to a long backboard and begin the secondary survey.
5. Perform secondary survey, including neurological examination and splinting of fractures.
6. Transport with continuous monitoring.

Once you have done the first four steps, you begin evaluation of the head injury. It is very important that this be recorded because the eventual treatment is often dictated by changes in the observed signs.

Primary Assessment

I. **Level of consciousness**

Level of consciousness is the most sensitive measure of brain function. Decreased level of consciousness in a trauma victim is usually due to head injury, shock, or drugs (usually alcohol). As a practical rule, you should always expect the cause to be head injury or shock. Use simple terms so that everyone can understand. The AVPU method is quite adequate.

A   Patient is alert.

V   Patient responds to vocal stimuli (any response to talking or shouting in his ear).

P   Patient responds to painful stimuli (pressure over sternum, or pinching fingers or toes).

U   Patient is unresponsive.

For a patient in a coma, the Glascow coma scale is simple and easy to use and has good prognostic value as to eventual outcome. It is included at the end of the chapter.

II. **Vital signs**

These are extremely important in following the course of head trauma. They may indicate changes in pressure within the skull. You should record vital signs every 5 minutes if possible.

A. *Blood pressure:* Increasing intracranial pressure causes an increased blood pressure; remember that other things do also (fear, pain, hypertension).

B. *Pulse:* Increasing intracranial pressure causes the pulse to decrease.

C. *Respiration:* Increasing intracranial pressure causes the respiratory rate to decrease. There may be several other respiratory patterns, depending on the injury. As a terminal event, the patient may

Comparison of Vital Signs in Shock and Head Injury

	Shock	Head Injury with Increasing Intracranial Pressure
Blood pressure	↓	↑
Pulse	↑	↓
Respiration	↑	↓
Level of consciousness	↓	↓

Figure 8–8.

show central neurogenic hyperventilation (rapid noisy respiration). Respiration is affected by so many factors (e.g., fear, hysteria, chest injuries, spinal cord injuries, diabetes) that it is not as useful an indicator as the other signs in monitoring the course of head injury.

Secondary Assessment

All patients with head or facial injuries must be thought of as also having cervical spine injuries until proven otherwise. Stabilization of the cervical spine begins with airway and breathing evaluation.

Once the primary survey is completed and recorded, begin with the head and quickly, but carefully, examine for obvious injuries such as lacerations or depressed or open skull fractures. The size of lacerations is often misjudged because of the difficulty in finding them in hair matted with blood. Feel the scalp with your fingers for obvious unstable areas of the skull. If none are present, apply a pressure dressing or hold direct pressure to stop the bleeding. A fracture of the base of the skull may be indicated by bleeding from the ear or nose, bruising behind the ear (Battle's sign) and/or swelling and discoloration around both eyes (raccoon eyes).

Pupils: The pupils are controlled by the third cranial nerve. This nerve takes a long course through the skull and is easily compressed by brain swelling. It thus serves as an early indicator of increasing pressure in the skull. A pupil that is dilated because of brain injury will always be associated with a decreased level of consciousness. If the victim is completely alert, you can be reasonably sure that a dilated pupil is *not* from brain injury. If both pupils are dilated and do not react to light, the patient probably has a brainstem injury and the prognosis is grim. If the pupils are dilated but still react to light, the injury is probably still reversible, so every effort should be made to get the patient quickly to a facility capable of treating a head injury. A dilated pupil on one side that remains reactive to light may be the earliest sign of increasing intracranial pressure. The development of a unilaterally dilated pupil while you are observing the patient is a sign of extreme emergency—in other words, load and go!

Fluttering eyelids are often seen with hysteria. Slow lid closure (like a curtain falling) is not seen with hysteria.

The doll's eyes test is a test of brainstem function. *It is never performed in the field! To do so might cause permanent paralysis!*

Extremities: Note sensation and motor function in the extremities. Can the patient feel you touch his hands and feet? Can he wiggle his fingers and toes?

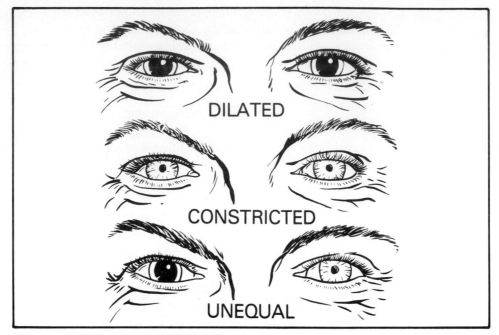

Figure 8-9.   Pupils of the eyes.

If the victim is unconscious, note his response to pain. If he withdraws or localizes to the pinching of his fingers and toes, he has intact sensation and motor function. This is a sign of normal or only minimally impaired cortical function.

Both decorticate posturing (arms flexed, legs extended) and decerebrate posturing (arms and legs extended) are ominous signs of deep cerebral hemispheric or upper brainstem injury. Flaccid paralysis usually means spinal cord injury.

Decisions on management of the head trauma patient are made on the basis of changes in all of these different signs. You are establishing the baseline from which later judgments must be made: record your observations.

Management of the Head Trauma Victim

You can provide important early treatment for the head trauma victim in the field. It is most important to make a rapid assessment and then begin oxygen and hyperventilation. Rapidly transport the victim to a facility capable of treating head trauma. The important points of management in the field are these:

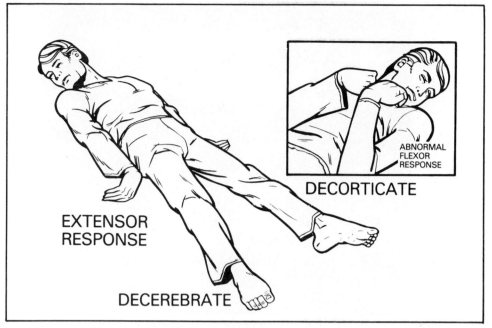

Figure 8–10.   Decorticate and decerebrate posturing.

1. Secure the airway and begin hyperventilation with high-flow oxygen. The brain does not tolerate hypoxia, so good ventilation is mandatory. The head injury patient should be hyperventilated. This decreases pressure in the skull. Be sure the neck is securely immobilized. Use a blanket roll or other padded immobilization device (not sandbags).

2. During transport, record baseline observations: This includes recording the level of consciousness, vital signs, pupils, and extremity movement and sensation. If the patient develops signs of shock, look for another cause.

3. Frequently monitor and record the observations listed above.

Potential Problems

1. *Convulsions:* Head trauma, especially intracranial hemorrhage, may cause convulsions. Be sure that the victim is well secured to the spine board.

2. *Vomiting:* A patient with head trauma almost always vomits. You must remain alert to this to prevent aspiration. Have suction available and be ready to log-roll him on his side (maintaining immobilization of the cervical spine).

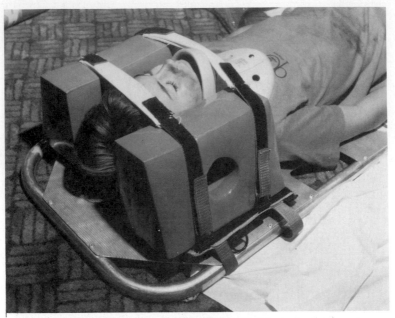

Figure 8-11.   Padded immobilization device.

3. *Rapidly deteriorating condition:* A patient who shows rapid deterioration of signs should be rapidly transported to improve changes for survival. Call ahead so that a neurosurgeon can be available and the operating room prepared by the time you arrive at the hospital. Developing rapid field response will not make up for time lost getting the appropriate doctor to the hospital. *Call early.*

4. *Shock:* If shock develops, think "Spinal cord injury or bleeding into chest or abdomen."

Summary of Management of the Patient with Decreased LOC

1. Stabilize the neck.
2. Secure and maintain the airway.
3. Give oxygen.
4. Hyperventilate (>24 breaths per minute).
5. Transport without delay.
6. Record baseline vital signs, observations of pupils, and neurological examination.
7. Continuously monitor and record.

Glasgow Coma Scale

This is a simple way to evaluate and monitor the patient who is in coma from *head trauma.* It has good value in predicting the outcome. There are three components. Score by the best response.

Eye Opening
Spontaneous 4
To voice 3
To pain 2
None 1

Verbal Response
Oriented...................... 5
Confused 4
Curses........................ 3
Incomprehensible
    sounds...................... 2
None 1

Motor Response
Obeys 6
Localizes..................... 5
Withdraws.................... 4
Flexion
    (decorticate)............... 3
Extension
    (decerebrate).............. 2
None 1

Total Scores
8 or better . . .
    94% favorable outcome
5, 6, 7 . . .
    50% favorable outcome
    (children 90%)
3 and 4 . . .
    10% favorable outcome
5, 6, 7 who drop a grade . . .
    100% unfavorable
    outcome
5, 6, 7 who improve to
    greater than 7 . . .
    80% favorable outcome

Figure 8–12.

Chapter 9

ABDOMINAL TRAUMA

Abdominal trauma may be blunt or penetrating. Most victims will live long enough to arrive at the hospital; most deaths occur because of a delay in diagnosis of intra-abdominal injury requiring surgery (surgery in the first 12 hours: 12 percent mortality; surgery after 12 hours: 50 percent mortality). Only a small percentage of multiple trauma victims will have clinical signs and symptoms of abdominal injury (less than 3 percent in one study), but about 40 percent of these victims will have abdominal injuries severe enough to require surgery. Thus it is important to have a high index of suspicion for abdominal injury and to record any changes noted during evaluation and transport. Those victims who have major abdominal vascular injuries bleed to death quickly.

Anatomy

The abdomen contains the liver, spleen, pancreas, stomach, intestines, aorta, inferior vena cava, kidneys, bladder, lower vertebral column, pelvis, and the spinal cord. In the woman there are also the ovaries and uterus. For practical purposes, the abdomen is divided into three areas for evaluation.

Intrathoracic Abdomen

This area is underneath the lower ribs and thus difficult to palpate. The liver, stomach, spleen, and diaphragm are found here. Injury to the lower ribs is often associated with injury to the underlying organs—especially the liver and spleen.

True Abdomen

This is the area we commonly think of as the "abdomen." It contains the large and small intestines, the bladder, and for practical purposes, the pelvis. Although this area is easier to examine, it is often difficult to decide between contusions of the abdominal wall and injury to the contents of the abdomen.

Retroperitoneal Abdomen

This is the area behind the posterior peritoneum. It contains the pancreas and part of the duodenum, the abdominal aorta, inferior vena cava, kidneys, uterus, and for practical purposes, the lower vertebral column and spinal cord. This area is very difficult to examine, and diagnosis of injuries often requires sophisticated procedures.

Figure 9–1. Intrathoracic abdomen.

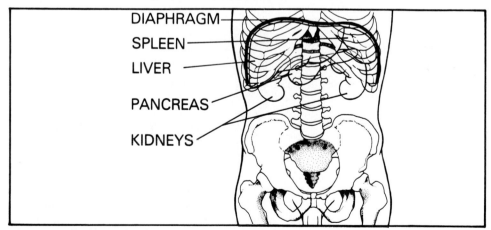

DIAPHRAGM
SPLEEN
LIVER
PANCREAS
KIDNEYS

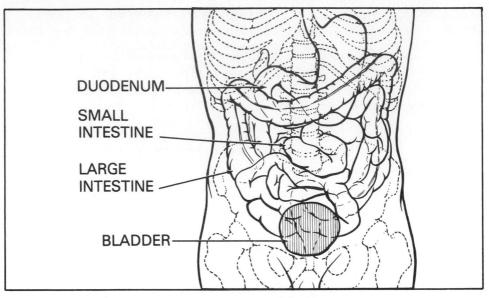

Figure 9–2.   True abdomen.

Figure 9–3.   Retroperitoneal abdomen.

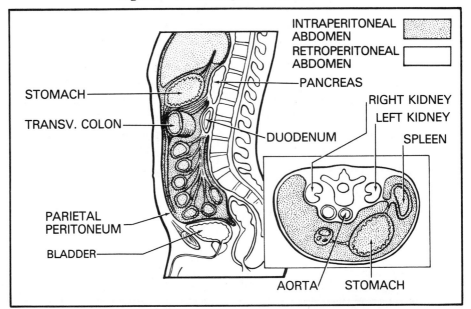

Types of Injuries

Penetrating Injuries

These can be from stab wounds or gunshot wounds. Injuries include the following:

1. Injuries to vessels, causing hemorrhage
2. Injuries to organs, causing hemorrhage
3. Injuries to organs, causing organ failure
4. Perforation of intestines
5. Protrusion of intestines through the wound

The first two types of injuries may present immediately as hypovolemic shock or may not show up for hours. The second two types of injuries will usually not present themselves for hours or even days. Protrusion of intestines through the wound is, of course immediately obvious. Thus, in penetrating injuries of the abdomen, your immediate concern is development of hypovolemic shock. Remember that a patient with a gunshot wound or stab wound (depending on the length of the instrument) of the chest, flank, or back may have an injury in the abdomen.

Blunt Abdominal Trauma

This injury can be from direct compression of the abdomen, with fracture of solid organs and blowout of hollow organs, or from deceleration, with tearing of organs or their blood vessels. As in penetrating injuries, the immediate danger to the patient is severe hemorrhage. A blunt abdominal injury frequently does not present with impressive signs and symptoms early, so you must keep a high index of suspicion to be prepared for the development of hemorrhagic shock.

Evaluation and Stabilization of the Patient with a Suspected Abdominal Injury

I. **Observation and history**
   Develop the habit of critically appraising the scene of an accident to predict what types of injuries could have been sustained: Poorly ad-

justed seat belts can cause rupture of the bladder or diaphragm, the steering wheel can cause abdominal as well as chest injuries, and broken windows or door knobs can injure the abdomen or chest. Accidents in which the car has flipped over can result in injury to any system. If a stab wound occurred, how long was the instrument? If the patient was shot, was the trajectory of the bullet up or down? Your observation and questions at the scene can be extremely helpful to the physician who must evaluate the patient at the emergency department.

II.   **Examination**

First follow the ABCs. The abdomen is generally examined during the MAST survey or the secondary survey. Use standard (but modified) look, listen, and feel examination.

A.   *Look:* Look at the front, back, and sides of the abdomen. The back is examined as you log-roll the patient onto the backboard. Notice if the abdomen is distended or if any bruises, abrasions, lacerations, puncture wounds, or protruding intestines are present.

B.   *Do NOT listen:* Listening for bowel sounds in the field is probably a waste of the golden hour. It can be done after the victim arrives at the hospital.

C.   *Feel:* Gently feel the anterior and posterior abdomen and record tenderness or masses. Do not worry about trying to decide on specific injuries; that can be done at the emergency department. If there are any indications of abdominal injury, you must be prepared to treat hemorrhagic shock.

III.   **Stabilization**

A.   Protruding intestines should be covered with sterile dressings moistened with saline or water. Do not attempt to push the intestines back into the abdomen. You cannot use the abdominal section of the antishock trousers if intestines are protruding.

B.   Any patient with possible abdominal injury should have the antishock garment applied, but not inflated. The vital signs and clinical condition should be carefully watched; if signs of shock appear, the garment should be inflated.

Important Points to Remember

1.   In the first hours after trauma, a tightly distended abdomen means massive intraabdominal bleeding. This patient must have the antishock garment and rapid transport. You should call ahead to see that the surgeon and operating room are ready when you arrive.

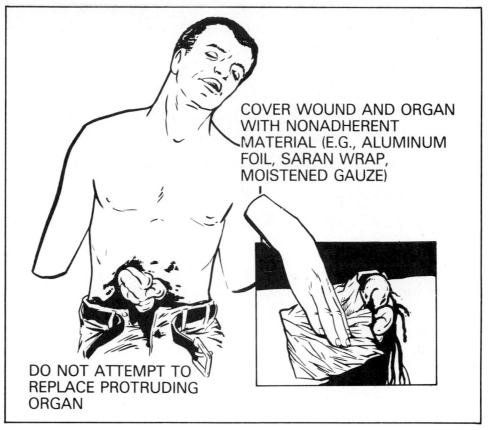

COVER WOUND AND ORGAN WITH NONADHERENT MATERIAL (E.G., ALUMINUM FOIL, SARAN WRAP, MOISTENED GAUZE)

DO NOT ATTEMPT TO REPLACE PROTRUDING ORGAN

Figure 9–4.   Protruding intestines.

2. A patient with hypotension, pallor, and tachycardia but no external injuries has bleeding into the abdomen or chest until proven otherwise.

3. Any gunshot or stab wound of the chest, flank, or back may have penetrated the abdomen.

4. Most deaths from abdominal trauma occur because of delayed diagnosis of a possible surgical abdomen. If your observation of the scene makes you think abdominal injury could have occurred, tell the receiving physician.

Chapter 10

EXTREMITY TRAUMA

Fractures, dislocations, and soft tissue injuries of the extremities are often the most dramatic injuries apparent when first examining a victim. Such injuries, although often disabling, are rarely immediately life threatening. You must keep in mind the importance of treating life-threatening injuries first. Thus airway, breathing, circulation, bleeding, and treatment of critical trauma situations precede splinting of fractures.

Hemorrhagic shock is a potential danger of very few musculoskeletal injuries. Only direct lacerations of arteries or fractures of the pelvis or femur are commonly associated with sufficient bleeding to cause shock. Injuries to nerves, arteries, or veins in the extremities are the most common complications of fractures and dislocations. Thus evaluation of sensation (feeling) and circulation (pulses, color) distal to the fractures is very important.

Injuries

A. *Fractures:* Fractures may be open (compound) with the broken end of the bone still protruding or having once protruded through the skin, or they may be closed (simple) with no communication to the outside. Fractured bone ends are extremely sharp and are quite dangerous to all the tissues that surround the bone. Since nerves and arteries frequently travel near the bone, across the flexor side of joints, or very near the skin in the hands and feet, they are frequently injured by lacerations due to bone fragments or by pressure due to swelling or hematomas. Closed fractures can be just as dangerous as open fractures. Significant amounts of blood can be lost into injured soft tissue. A fractured femur can cause the loss of 2 units of blood (a unit is about a pint), and a fractured pelvis can cause the loss of 1 unit for every fracture (up to 20 units). Pelvic fractures that lacerate the large pelvic vessels can cause fatal hemorrhage. Remember, multiple fractures can cause life-threatening hemorrhage without any external blood

Figure 10–1. Classification of fractures.

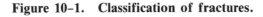

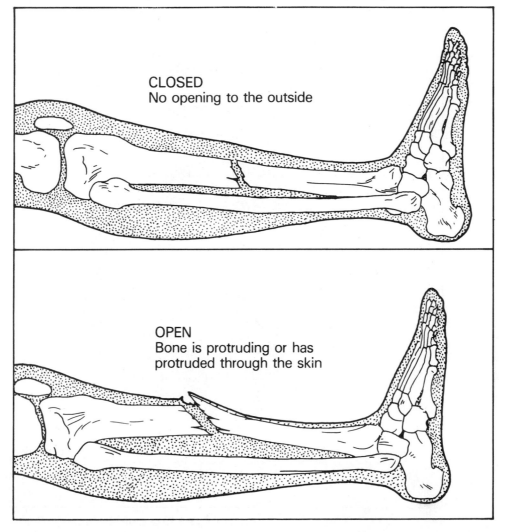

CLOSED
No opening to the outside

OPEN
Bone is protruding or has protruded through the skin

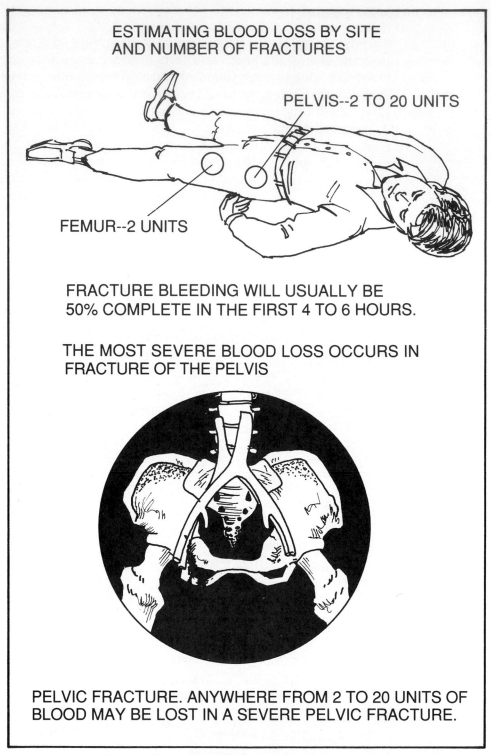

ESTIMATING BLOOD LOSS BY SITE
AND NUMBER OF FRACTURES

PELVIS--2 TO 20 UNITS

FEMUR--2 UNITS

FRACTURE BLEEDING WILL USUALLY BE
50% COMPLETE IN THE FIRST 4 TO 6 HOURS.

THE MOST SEVERE BLOOD LOSS OCCURS IN
FRACTURE OF THE PELVIS

PELVIC FRACTURE. ANYWHERE FROM 2 TO 20 UNITS OF
BLOOD MAY BE LOST IN A SEVERE PELVIC FRACTURE.

Figure 10–2. Internal blood loss from fractures.

loss. Open fractures add the dangers of external hemorrhage and contamination of the wound with bacteria.

B. *Dislocations:* Joint dislocations are extremely painful injuries. They are almost always easy to identify because of distortion of the normal anatomy. Major joint dislocations, although not life threatening, are often true emergencies because of pressure on nerves and arteries which can, if not treated quickly, lead to loss of a limb. It is very important to check for sensation, pallor, and pulses distal to major joint dislocations. The normal rule is to splint joint injuries in the position that you find them. Pad and splint the extremity in the most comfortable position and rapidly transport the patient to a facility that has orthopedic care available.

C. *Amputations:* These are disabling and sometimes life-threatening injuries. The stump should be covered with moist sterile dressings and an elastic wrap. If bleeding cannot be controlled with pressure, a tourniquet may be used. If you can find the amputated part, bring it with you, but do not give the patient false hopes about reimplantation.

Figure 10–3. Transportation of amputated part. If ice and time are available, seal part in small container and place this in larger container of ice and water. Do *not* use dry ice. Do *not* place amputated part directly on ice. If no ice is available, *place part in plastic bag* and *seal* so that the part will not lose moisture. Do *not* wrap part in moistened dressing.

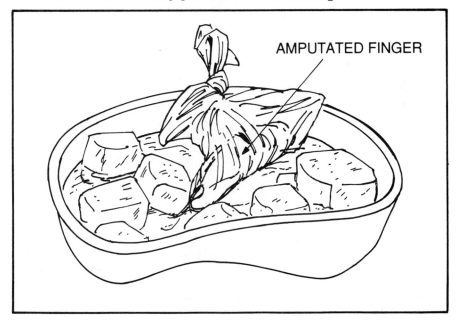

Situations in which reimplantation is usually not done are:
1. Patients with other major injuries
2. Patients over the age of 40 years
3. Avulsion (torn off) injuries
4. Crush injuries
5. Amputations involving the lower extremities
Small amputated parts should be sealed in a small plastic bag. If ice is available, place the bag in a larger bag or container containing ice and water. Do not use ice alone and never use dry ice. Cooling the part will increase the viability from 4 to 6 hours to about 18 hours. It is important to bring amputated parts even if reimplantation is not feasible. Some of the part may be used in the repair.

D. *Wounds:* Cover wounds with a sterile dressing and bandage. Bleeding can be stopped with pressure dressings or air splints. Tourniquets are almost never needed.

E. *Neurovascular injuries:* The nerves and major vessels generally run side by side and thus may be injured together. Loss of circulation and/or sensation can be due to swelling, disruption by missiles or broken bone ends, or compression by the bone fragments. Extremity

Figure 10–4.   Palpation of radial pulse.

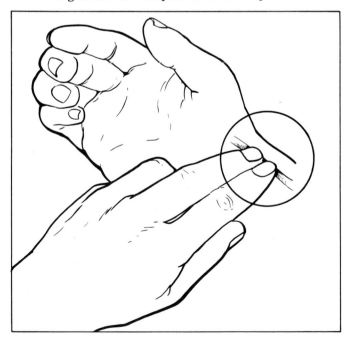

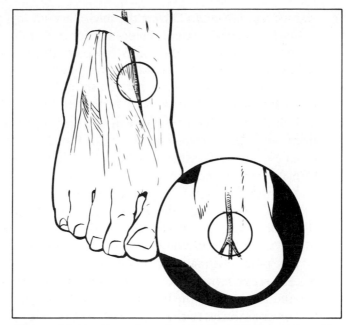

Figure 10–5. Location of posterior tibial and dorsalis pedis pulses.

pulses and sensation are always checked before and after straightening of fractures and after application of splints or traction.

F. *Sprains and strains:* These injuries cannot be differentiated from fractures in the field. Treat them as if they are fractures.

G. *Impaled objects:* Do not remove them. Apply padding and transport the patient with the object in place. Any motion outside the body is transmitted within the tissue where the end of the object may lacerate or harm sensitive structures. Removing the object may cause bleeding that is impossible to control. The cheek of the face is an exception to this rule. Another exception is the patient in cardiac arrest with an impaled object in the chest preventing CPR.

Assessment and Management

A. *History:* This is especially important in extremity trauma. It is important to note the apparent mechanisms of injury and the position and condition of the extremity when you first arrive. No time should be wasted trying to obtain a verbal history until airway, breathing, and circulatory status is clearly established. In the conscious patient, the history is obtained while performing the secondary survey.

B. *Assessment (general):* During the secondary survey, you should quickly palpate (feel) each extremity, looking for deformity and areas of spasm or tenderness. Check the joints for pain and movement. Check and record distal pulses and sensation. Crepitation or grating of bone ends is a definite sign of fracture, but you should not attempt to demonstrate it since you would be causing further injury to the soft tissue.

C. *Management (general):* Proper management of fractures and dislocations will reduce serious complications and may well prevent the loss of an extremity. Treatment in the field is directed at proper immobilization of the injured part by use of a splint.

   1. *Purpose of splinting:* The objective is to prevent motion in the broken bone ends, thereby preventing further damage to muscles, nerves, and blood vessels. Proper splinting also reduces pain.

   2. *When to use splinting:* There is no simple rule that will determine the precise sequence to follow in every trauma patient. In general, the more serious the trauma, the less time spent in the field with immobilization the better. The multiply traumatized patient with severe injuries to the trunk may have the lower extremities briefly examined (MAST survey) and splinted within a MAST suit almost

Figure 10-6. Reasons for splinting.

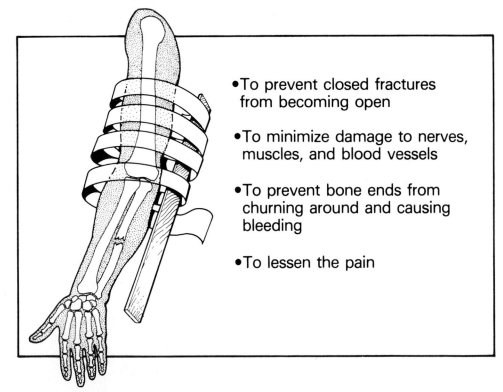

- To prevent closed fractures from becoming open

- To minimize damage to nerves, muscles, and blood vessels

- To prevent bone ends from churning around and causing bleeding

- To lessen the pain

immediately after the primary survey. This rapidly and effectively does what traction splints might be required to do and effectively saves very critical time. The patient who requires a "load and go" approach can be adequately stabilized by careful packaging on the long spine board. This does not mean that the EMT has no responsibility to identify and protect extremity fractures, but rather implies that some splinting can be done in the vehicle in route to the hospital. It is never appropriate to sacrifice time, which may be important in saving a life to prevent disability by immobilizing a limb.

3. *General rules of splinting*

   a. You must adequately visualize the injured part. Clothes must be cut off, not pulled off, unless there is only an isolated injury that presents no problem with maintaining immobilization.

   b. Check and record distal sensation and circulation before and after splinting. Check movement distal to the fracture if possible (e.g., ask the patient to wiggle his fingers or toes).

   c. If the extremity is severely angulated, you should apply gentle traction in an attempt to straighten it. If resistance is encountered, splint it in the angulated position.

Figure 10-7. Straightening angulated fractures.

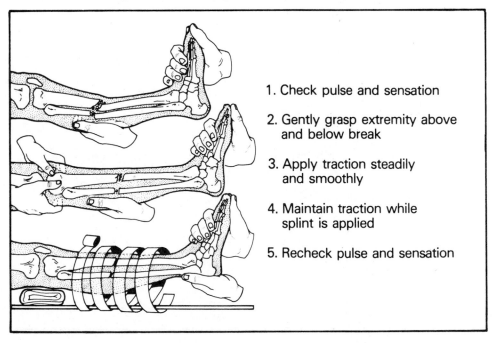

1. Check pulse and sensation

2. Gently grasp extremity above and below break

3. Apply traction steadily and smoothly

4. Maintain traction while splint is applied

5. Recheck pulse and sensation

    d.   Open wounds should be covered with sterile dressings before you apply the splint.

    e.   Use a splint that will immobilize one joint above and below the injury.

    f.   Pad the splint well.

    g.   Do not attempt to push bone ends back under the skin. When you apply traction, if the bone end retracts back into the wound, allow it to do so but be sure you notify the receiving physician.

    h.   Splint all injuries before moving the patient unless a life-threatening situation prevents it.

    i.   If in doubt, splint.

4.   *Types of splints*

    a.   *Rigid splint:* This type of splint can be made from many different materials, such as cardboard, plastic, metal, or wood. It should be padded well and should always extend one joint above and below the fracture.

    b.   *Soft splint:* This type includes air splints, vacuum splints, pillows, and slings and swathes.

Figure 10–8a.   Types of splints.

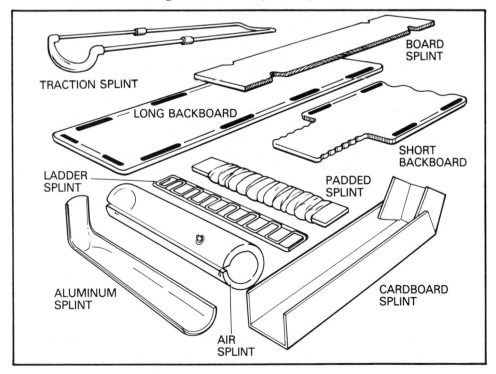

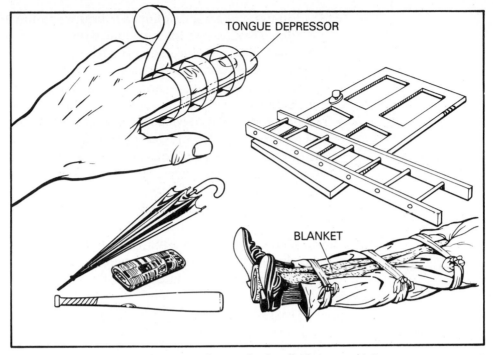

Figure 10–8b. Improvised splinting materials.

(1) Air splints are good for fractures of the lower arm and lower leg. They have the advantage of compression to stop bleeding and swelling in the area that they cover. You must blow these up by mouth (never a pump) until they give good support and yet can be easily dented with slight pressure from a fingertip. Remember that if they are applied in a cold environment, the pressure will increase as they warm up. The pressure also increases if they are applied on the ground and then the patient is transported by air. When you use air splints, you must constantly check the pressure to be sure that the splint is not getting too tight (or too loose—they often leak). There are two major disadvantages of air splints: You cannot monitor extremity pulses while they are applied, and the splints often stick to the skin and are painful to remove.

(2) Vacuum splints are excellent in that they can be molded to stabilize fractures in any position. Their only disadvantage is they are very bulky and can be a problem to store in the rescue vehicle.

(3) Pillows make good splints for injuries to the ankle or foot. They are also helpful along with a sling and swathe to stabilize a dislocated shoulder.

(4) Slings and swathes are excellent for injuries to the clavicle, shoulder, upper arm, elbow, and sometimes the forearm.

c. *Traction splint:* This device is designed for fractures of the lower extremities. It holds a fracture immobile by the application of a steady pull on the extremity. The most common are the Thomas, Sager, Hare, and Klippel splints. They are used to immobilize fractures of the femur and proximal tibia and fibula, and they work by applying countertraction to the ischium and groin. They must be padded and applied with care to prevent excessive pressure on the genitalia. You must also use care in applying the hitching device to the foot and ankle so as not to interfere with circulation.

D. *Management (specific injuries)*

1. *Spine:* This is covered elsewhere in the book but included here to remind you that if there is any chance of spinal injury, proper immobilization must be done to prevent lifelong paralysis or even death from a spinal cord injury. Remember, a fall in which a victim lands on his feet may cause lumbar spine fracture.

Figure 10–9.   Spine board with rigid extrication collar and padded immobilization device. Collars do not give adequate lateral support—use padded immobilization device also.

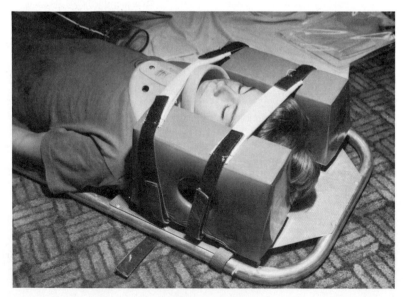

2. *Pelvis:* While the pelvis is not an extremity, it is practical to incude injuries to it here. These injuries are usually caused by motor vehicle accidents or by falls from a height. There is always the potential for serious hemorrhage in pelvic fractures, so shock should be expected and prepared for. There is a high (10 percent) incidence of injuries to the bladder or urethra associated with pelvic fractures, but there is little you can do for these injuries in the field. A patient with a pelvic injury should be transported on a spine board. Pelvic fractures can be associated with severe bleeding; therefore, antishock garmet should be used to splint and to tamponade bleeding.

3. *Femur:* The femur is the longest and heaviest bone in the body. It usually fractures at midshaft and often is an open fracture. There is usually significant bleeding by the heavy muscles of the thigh. Bilateral femur fractures can be associated with loss of 50 percent of the circulating blood volume, so be prepared for development of shock. Use a traction splint. If there is no angulation or severe shortening of the leg, you may use the antishock garment alone as a splint. If a traction splint is to be used with the antishock garment, apply the splint after the garment is applied, but before it is inflated.

Figure 10-10a. Applying a traction splint.

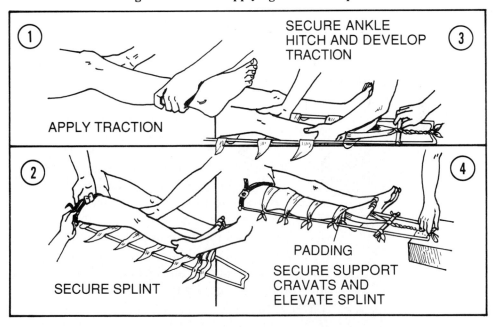

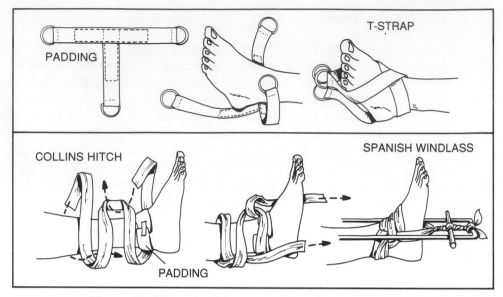

Figure 10-10b. Applying a traction hitch to the ankle.

4. *Hip*

    a. Hip fractures are usually in the neck of the femur. These are probably the most common fractures in elderly people. The neck of the femur is very short and is completely surrounded by strong ligaments; thus there is not much movement of the bone ends and little bleeding occurs. Because of the strength of the ligamentous structures, the fractured hip may still bear weight, but do not be fooled into thinking a fracture does not exist because the patient has walked with help. A traction splint is not necessary. The uninjured leg can be used to splint the fractured one. Hip fractures often refer pain to the knee, so always think of hip fracture when an elderly person falls and complains of knee pain only.

    b. Hip dislocation is a different story. Most hip dislocations are the result of car accidents in which the knee strikes the dashboard, forcing the hip out the posterior side of the joint. This is an orthopedic emergency and requires reduction as soon as possible to prevent sciatic nerve injury or necrosis of the femoral head. The hip will usually be flexed, and the victim will not be able to tolerate having the leg straightened. A hip dislocation should be supported in the most comfortable position by use of pillows and the uninjured leg. Transport the patient rapidly to a facility where orthopedic care is available.

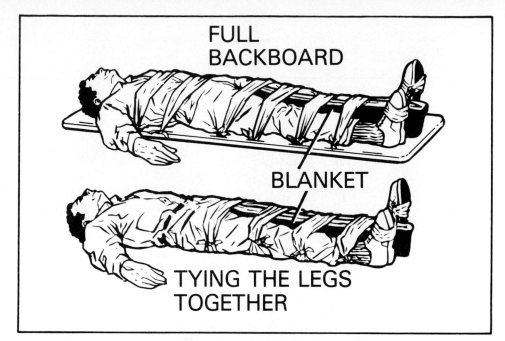

FULL
BACKBOARD

BLANKET

TYING THE LEGS
TOGETHER

Figure 10–11. Hip fracture.

Figure 10–12. Mechanism of posterior dislocation of the hip. "Down and Under."

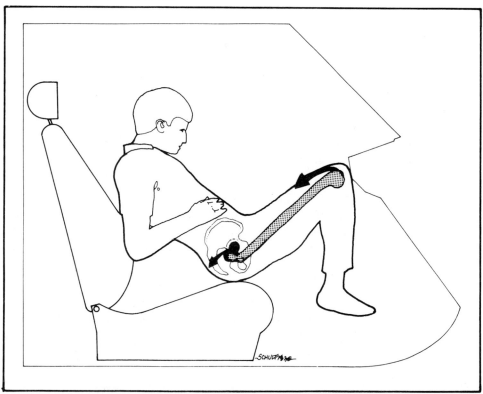

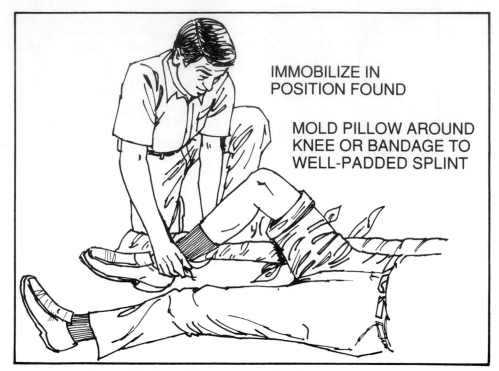

IMMOBILIZE IN POSITION FOUND

MOLD PILLOW AROUND KNEE OR BANDAGE TO WELL-PADDED SPLINT

Figure 10–13.   Splinting posterior dislocation of the hip.

5. *Knee:* Fractures or dislocations here are serious because the arteries are bound down above and below the knee and are often disrupted if the joint dislocates. About 50 percent of knee dislocations have associated vascular injuries, and many require amputation. Prompt reduction of knee dislocation is mandatory. You should apply *gentle* traction; many will easily reduce. Do *not* apply traction with a traction splint; you may tear the arteries in the knee. If there is resistance to straightening the knee, splint it in the most comfortable position and transport the patient rapidly to a facility where orthopedic care is available. This is another true orthopedic emergency.

6. *Tibia/fibula:* Fractures of the lower leg are frequently the results of motorcycle or automobile accidents. They are often open and often have significant internal and/or external blood loss. Fractures of the upper tibia may be immobilized with a traction splint. Fractures of the lower leg may be splinted with a rigid splint or air splint.

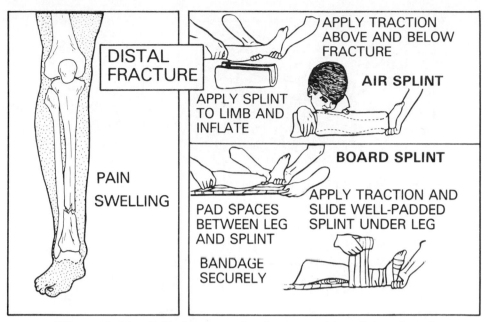

Figure 10–14.   Splinting lower leg fractures. Air splint or board splint.

7. *Clavicle:* This is the bone through which the upper extremity (arm) attaches to the central skeleton. It is the site of one of the most frequent fractures but rarely causes problems even though the subclavian artery and vein lie just beneath it. It is best immobilized in the field with a sling and swathe.

8. *Shoulder:* Most shoulder injuries are either a dislocation of the joint, a separation of the acromioclavicular joint, or fracture of the upper humerus. A sling and swathe usually provides the best immobilization. Dislocated shoulders are very painful and often require a pillow between the arm and body to hold the upper arm at the most comfortable position.

9. *Elbow:* It is often difficult to tell whether there is fracture or dislocation; both can be serious because of the danger of neurovascular injury. Elbow injuries should always be splinted in the most comfortable position and the patient rapidly transported for treatment. Do not attempt to straighten or apply traction to an elbow injury.

10. *Forearm and wrist:* This is a very common fracture, usually as a result of a fall on the outstretched arm. It is best immobilized

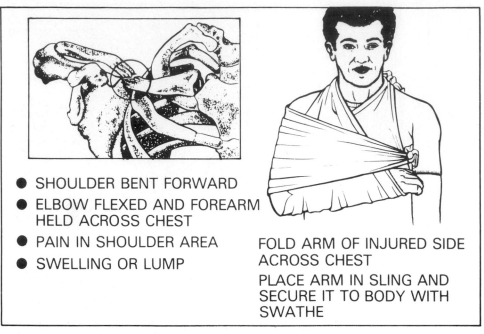

- SHOULDER BENT FORWARD
- ELBOW FLEXED AND FOREARM HELD ACROSS CHEST
- PAIN IN SHOULDER AREA
- SWELLING OR LUMP

FOLD ARM OF INJURED SIDE ACROSS CHEST

PLACE ARM IN SLING AND SECURE IT TO BODY WITH SWATHE

Figure 10–15.   Fractured clavicle.

Figure 10–16.   Dislocated shoulder.

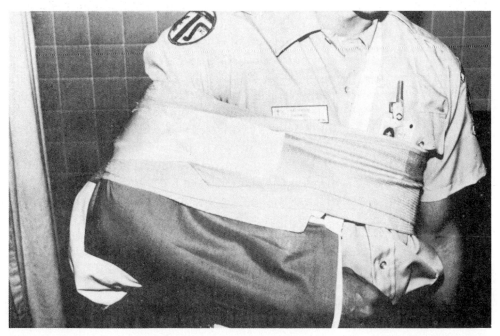

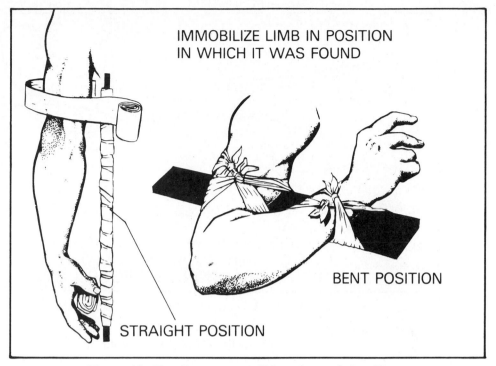

Figure 10–17.   Fractures or dislocations of the elbow.

with a rigid splint or an air splint. If a rigid splint is used, put a roll of gauze in the hand to hold it in the position of function.

11. *Hand or foot:* Industrial accidents involving the hand or foot often produce multiple open fractures and even avulsions. These injuries are often disabling and gruesome appearing but are usually not associated with life-threatening hemorrhage. A pillow is usually support enough for these injuries.

Important Points to Remember

1. Be alert to mechanisms of injury so that you will know what fractures to suspect.
2. Visualize the injured part.
3. Be prepared for hemorrhagic shock in those fractures associated with significant bleeding.
4. Always record sensation and circulation initially and after any manipulation or splinting.

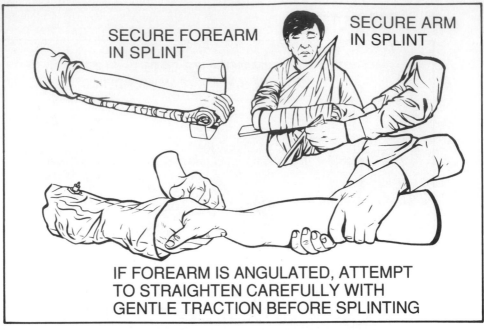

SECURE FOREARM IN SPLINT

SECURE ARM IN SPLINT

IF FOREARM IS ANGULATED, ATTEMPT TO STRAIGHTEN CAREFULLY WITH GENTLE TRACTION BEFORE SPLINTING

Figure 10–18.   Fractures of the forearm and wrist.

Figure 10–19.   Fracture of the ankle or foot.

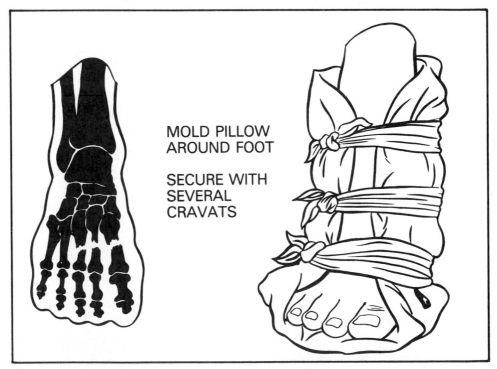

MOLD PILLOW AROUND FOOT

SECURE WITH SEVERAL CRAVATS

5. Pad splints well.
6. Immobilize one joint above and below the fracture.
7. Splint before moving unless the patient has a life-threatening condition.
8. If in doubt, splint.
9. Do not waste time. Be fast but be careful.
10. In critical situations splinting should be done in the ambulance or at the hospital. Get the victim on a spine board and transport.

Chapter 11

BURNS

A burn is an injury to tissue caused by direct thermal injury, exposure to a caustic chemical, or contact with an electrical current. Each year approximately 100,000 people require hospitalization for burns, and 12,000 die as the result of fires.

Anatomy and Physiology

The skin is made up of two layers: the epidermis and the dermis. The epidermis or top layer of the skin serves primarily as a protective layer for the deeper structures. The dermis or deeper layer of the skin contains the hair follicles, sweat glands, oil glands, and sensory fibers for pain, touch, pressure, and temperature. Underneath the dermis is a layer of connective tissue and fat deposits called the subcutaneous tissue.

The skin acts as an envelope to seal the body's fluids inside and germs outside. It is also an organ for sensation and temperature regulation and provides a flexible, mechanical, protective coat for the body.

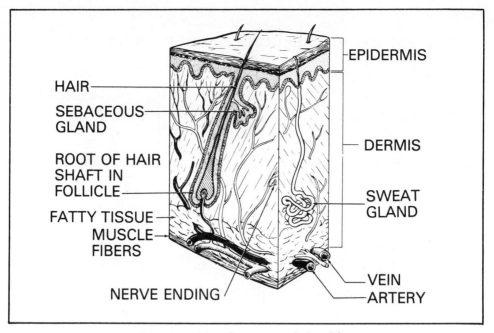

Figure 11–1.   Structure of the skin.

Pathophysiology

When heat or caustic chemicals are applied to the skin, the layers are destroyed. The severity of the injury depends on the depth of the burn and the surface area involved as well as on associated injuries.

A first-degree or superficial partial-thickness burn involves only the epidermal layer. The skin is inflamed and tender and may peel in a few days, but it requires no treatment and heals without scarring.

A second-degree or deep partial-thickness burn involves the epidermis and part of the dermis but spares the deeper structures in the dermis from which new cells grow to form a new dermis and epidermis. These burns are painful, have either blisters or open weeping areas, and can lose a significant amount of fluid. They usually heal within 14 to 21 days without scarring as long as infection does not develop.

A third-degree or full-thickness burn destroys the epidermis, dermis, and often even the subcutaneous or deeper layers. These burns are white or charred and have a hard, leathery feel. All sensation is lost because the sensory organs are destroyed. They are painful only around the edges, where they taper into

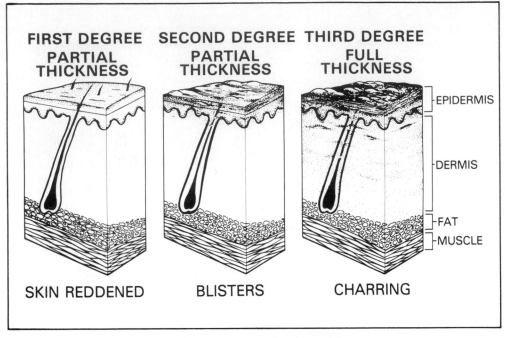

Figure 11–2.   Classification of burns.

partial-thickness burns. These burns heal by scar tissue formation. During healing the skin fails to function as a protective barrier to fluid loss or bacteria.

Burn deaths usually occur due to smoke inhalation, hypovolemic shock, or overwhelming infection.

Types of Burns

A.   *Thermal:* Injury to the tissue is caused directly by heat. This may not only injure the skin, but if the victim inhales the flames, may cause injury to the upper airway as well. The upper airway filters, humidifies, and warms or cools the air we breathe. It performs this function so well that flames, even when breathed into the mouth and nose, almost never cause thermal injury beyond the pharynx and upper trachea. This is because air does not hold heat well. It thus cools rapidly when breathed into the body. In contrast, water holds heat much better, so if steam is inhaled it causes thermal injury all the way to the alveoli. Upper airway burns cause swelling of the throat and trachea. This swelling is often enough to cause complete airway obstruction. These symptoms may not present themselves for hours after the initial in-

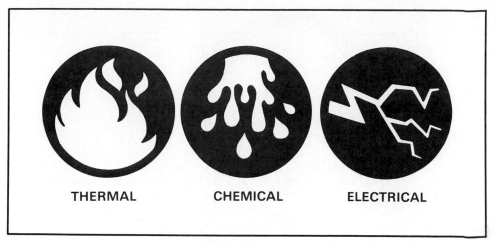

Figure 11–3.   Types of burns.

jury but may rapidly become life-threatening once they begin. All patients suspected of having thermal injury to the upper airway should be admitted to the hospital for close observation. At least 30% of patients hospitalized for burns have upper airway burns as well. These signs should alert you to the danger of upper airway burns:
1. Burns of the face
2. Singed eyebrows or nasal hairs
3. Burns in the mouth
4. Carbonaceous (sooty) sputum
5. History of unconsciousness while near a fire
6. History of being confined in a closed space while being burned

B. *Chemical:* Chemical burns cause tissue injury from damage by strong acids, alkalis, or other corrosive materials. The severity depends on the type of corrosive, the concentration of the solution, the area involved, and the time it remains in contact with the skin. Alkalis are generally worse than acids because they penetrate the skin more quickly and are more difficult to remove.

C. *Electrical:* An electrical burn may cause direct damage from the electrical current or death from fibrillation of the heart. Electricity also causes sudden contraction of the muscles, so there may be musculoskeletal injuries as well. Usually, high-voltage electrical burns have wounds of entrance and exit caused by the electric arc (temperature of 2500 degrees Celsius) with varying amounts of injury inside the body between the two points. Electrical current inside the body tends to follow the blood vessels and nerves, often destroying them as well as

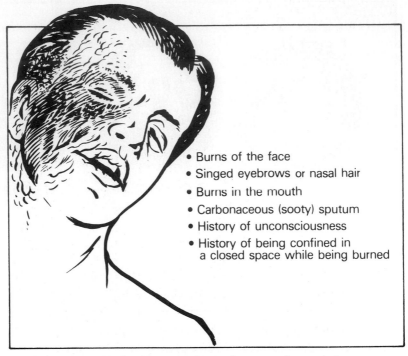

- Burns of the face
- Singed eyebrows or nasal hair
- Burns in the mouth
- Carbonaceous (sooty) sputum
- History of unconsciousness
- History of being confined in a closed space while being burned

Figure 11–4.   Danger signs of upper airway injury.

surrounding tissue. There may also be external thermal burns from the patient's clothing being ignited. It is impossible in the field to determine the amount of tissue damage because much of the damage may be inside the body. Thus all patients with electrical burns should be transported to the hospital for examination. Most will be admitted.

Associated Injuries

A.   *Smoke inhalation:* There are approximately 12,000 burn deaths each year. At least one-half of this number is due to smoke inhalation. There are over 200 toxic fumes produced from wood smoke and no one knows how many from synthetic products. Smoke inhalation damages the alveoli of the lungs, causing swelling and accumulation of fluid. This prevents air exchange and the victim smothers. The clinical picture is exactly like congestive heart failure. Most deaths occur at the scene from direct asphyxia (lack of oxygen), but many victims do not develop symptoms for up to 24 hours. All patients suspected of inhalation injury should be taken to the hospital for observation and tests. Situations in which you should suspect smoke inhalation:

1. Victims exposed to smoke in an enclosed space
2. Victims who were unconscious while exposed to smoke and fire
3. Victims with a cough after being exposed to smoke or fire
4. Victims short of breath after being exposed to smoke and fire
5. Victims with chest pain after being exposed to smoke or fire

B. *Carbon monoxide poisoning:* Fires in which there is not enough oxygen for complete combustion produce a gas called carbon monoxide. It is colorless, odorless, and tasteless. When breathed into the lungs, carbon monoxide has an affinity for hemoglobin that is over 200 times greater than that of oxygen. Thus carbon monoxide can saturate the hemoglobin molecules of the red cells so that they can no longer carry oxygen. The victim will die from hypoxia. Generally, no symptoms develop until the blood is about 20 percent saturated, at which time the victim complains of headache, nausea, and vomiting. At 30% satu-

Figure 11–5.   Danger signs of inhalation injury.

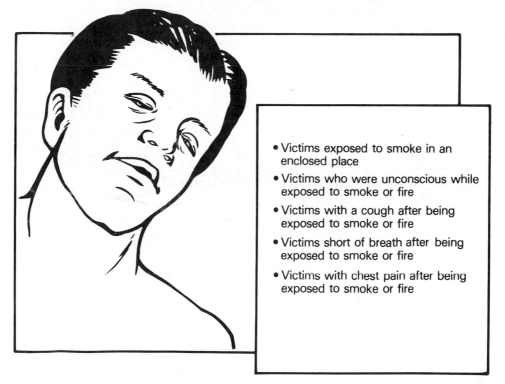

- Victims exposed to smoke in an enclosed place
- Victims who were unconscious while exposed to smoke or fire
- Victims with a cough after being exposed to smoke or fire
- Victims short of breath after being exposed to smoke or fire
- Victims with chest pain after being exposed to smoke or fire

ration he becomes confused, and at 40 to 50 percent saturation coma may occur. Convulsions and frequently death follow higher saturations. If the patient is simply removed from the source of the gas, it will take about 5 hours for the carbon monoxide to clear from the blood. Administration of 100 percent oxygen decreases this to about 90 minutes, and a hyperbaric oxygen chamber can decrease the time to less than 30 minutes. The carboxyhemoglobin molecule is bright red but the mythical "cherry red" victim of carbon monoxide poisoning has probably never been seen. Carbogen (95 percent oxygen and 5 percent carbon dioxide) was once given to miners in England as an antidote to carbon monoxide poisoning. The carbon *dioxide* caused rapid breathing, so the miners quickly exchanged oxygen for the carbon monoxide in their blood. Carbon dioxide is also a potent vasodilator, so the miners who breathed carbogen became "cherry red" from vasodilatation and hyperoxygenation. Thus the myth of the "cherry red" carbon monoxide victim began. The most common sources of carbon monoxide are automobile engines, poorly vented heating devices, and fires in closed spaces.

C. *Explosion injury:* Many fires are associated with explosions (e.g., propane gas explosions). Victims are often thrown some distance and may have fractures or internal injuries as well as burns. Chest injuries and inhalation injuries to the lungs are common in this type of accident.

Assessment of Burns

A. *History:* There are several things you should always record.
    1. What was the cause of the burn (an open flame, a chemical, a hot liquid)? It is very important to know the name and concentration of the chemical involved in chemical burns.
    2. Was an explosion involved? If so, you must expect and look for other injuries. Chest injuries are especially common here.
    3. Was the patient in a closed space, so that he may have inhaled smoke, steam, carbon monoxide, or flames?
    4. Was the patient unconscious?
    5. How long has it been since the burn occurred?
    6. What has already been done for the burn? Was anything applied?
    7. Past medical history: Does the patient have heart or lung disease or any other serious illness, such as diabetes?
    8. What medication is the patient taking?

B. *Depth of burn:* Estimate the depth from the appearance of the skin. Partial thickness burns are red or mottled, painful, and are blistered or swollen. Full-thickness burns are leathery and may be translucent or white. The surface is usually dry and nontender. It is impossible to estimate the depth of chemical and electrical burns initially.

C. *Extent of burn:* In the field, estimation of burn size need only be a "ballpark" figure. More precise determination of the size of the burn will be done at the hospital. What is important in the field is making the decision about which burned patients need to go to the hospital, and if a burn center is in your area, which patients need to go directly there.

1. *Rule of nines:* A reasonable estimate of burn size can be made by dividing the body into areas of 9 percent or 18 percent. The head is proportionally larger in a child. For estimating the size of multiple or irregular burns, you can use the guide that the palm of the patient's hand is equal to about 1 percent of his body surface area.

Figure 11–6.   Rule of nines.

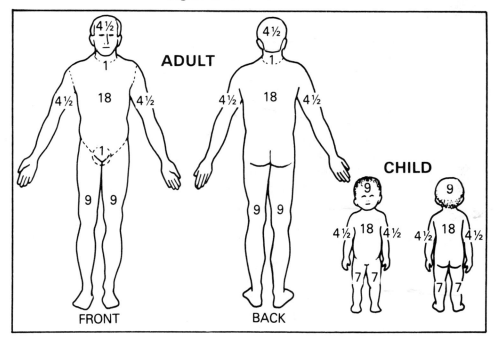

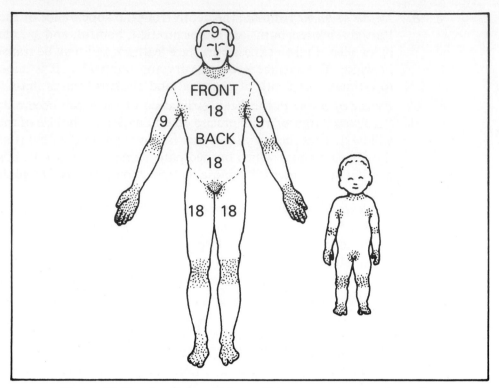

Figure 11–7.   Areas in which small burns are more serious. Second or third degree burns in these areas (shaded portions) should be treated in the hospital.

2. *Patients requiring hospital treatment*
    a. Any patient with a full-thickness burn of more than 2 percent of body surface area
    b. Any patient with a partial thickness burn of more than 10 percent of body surface area
    c. Significant burns of face, hands, feet, or genitalia
    d. Burns that involve flexion areas, such as neck, axilla, elbows, or knees
3. Patients that may need to be transported to a burn unit or burn center
    a. Full thickness burns exceeding 5 percent of body surface area
    b. Partial thickness burns exceeding 15 percent of body surface area
    c. Serious burns of hands, feet, genitalia, or perianal area
    d. Inhalation injury

      e. Significant burns about the face

      f. High-voltage electrical burns

      g. Burns associated with fractures or other major injuries

      h. Lesser burns in patients who are already sick

4. *As a general rule, all burns should be seen by a doctor.* Many partial-thickness burns have become full-thickness burns because of infection from lack of proper care.

Management of Burns

A. *Thermal burns*

1. Remove the victim from the fire or the fire from the victim. This is one of the few exceptions to the normal ABCs of resuscitation. In many instances the speedy removal of the patient (and yourself) to a safe area must take priority over all else. Even in these cases remember that, if possible, the neck and back should be stabilized until you are sure no injury to the spine exists. Obviously, there will be times when this is not possible. You must consider your own safety during a rescue—dead EMTs do not save lives.

2. Follow the ABCs of resuscitation.

3. Stop the burning process. Cool the burn with tap water (sterile water is not necessary) only until the temperature is the same as normal skin. This is to stop the burning process. Do not apply ice or ice water to extensive burns since this may cause hypothermia and worsen shock.

4. Remove clothing and jewelry. Cut around clothing that sticks to the skin.

5. Cover the burns with a clean sheet or sterile dressing. Do not apply any medications or ointments to the burn.

6. Complete the secondary survey.

7. If there is any chance of inhalation injury, give oxygen.

8. Transport the patient.

B. *Chemical burns*

1. The most important field treatment is removing or diluting the chemical agent. Irrigation with a neutral solution (water) must be carried out immediately. This should be done for 15 minutes at the scene. Use a water hose or shower: large volumes of water are needed. Do *not* try to neutralize acids with alkali or alkalis with acid; water is the only irrigant you should use. Clothes must be removed since they prevent removal of the chemical.

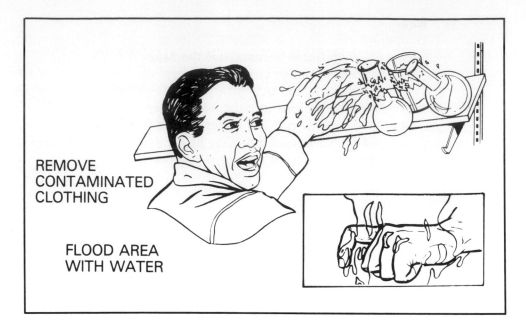

REMOVE
CONTAMINATED
CLOTHING

FLOOD AREA
WITH WATER

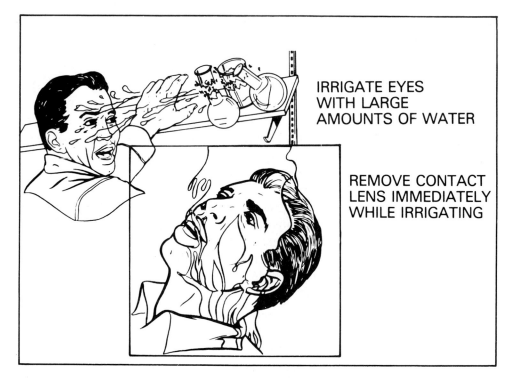

IRRIGATE EYES
WITH LARGE
AMOUNTS OF WATER

REMOVE CONTACT
LENS IMMEDIATELY
WHILE IRRIGATING

Figure 11–8a.   Chemical burns of the skin.
Figure 11–8b.   Chemical burns of the eye.

2. Dry lime or soda ash is a special case in that the addition of water causes a highly corrosive substance to form. The victim's clothes should be removed and the dry chemical brushed from his skin. If large volumes of water are available (hose or shower), the remainder of the chemical can be flushed away.

C. *Electrical burns:* Here again is an exception to the routine ABCs of resuscitation.

1. The first priority in electrical burns is determining whether the patient is still in contact with the electrical source. If he is, you must remove him from contact without becoming a victim yourself. Handling high-voltage electrical wires is extremely hazardous. Special training and special equipment are needed to deal with downed wires; you should never attempt to move wires with makeshift equipment. Tree limbs, pieces of wood, and even manila rope may conduct high-voltage electricity. Even firefighter's gloves and boots do not protect you in this situation. If possible, the handling of downed wires should be left to power company employees. It is better to turn off electricity at the source rather

Figure 11–9. Removal of high voltage electrical wires. *Do not* **try to remove wires with the safety equipment pictured (or with sticks) unless specially trained.** *Do* **turn off the electricity at the source or call the power company to remove the wires.**

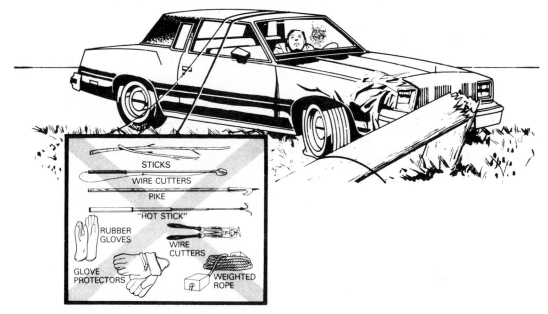

than move hot wires. An alternative is to develop a special training program with your local power company to learn how to use the special equipment needed to handle high-voltage wires.

2. Cardiac arrest is a frequent complication of electrocution, so cardiopulmonary resuscitation is often necessary; use standard resuscitation procedures once the patient is free from the source of electricity.

3. All electrical burns are critical burns until proven otherwise.

Important Points to Remember

1. Be alert at the scene: you must not become one of the victims.

2. Remember that burn victims often have other injuries as well.

3. Remember that inhalation injuries cause half of all burn deaths. The time to give oxygen is any time you think it might be needed.

4. Most burn patients, except victims of chemical burns, should be rapidly evaluated and transported. Chemical burns should be irrigated with water for 10 to 15 minutes unless other injuries dictate transport sooner.

Chapter 12

TRAUMA IN PREGNANCY

Trauma, specifically that sustained in automobile accidents, is the leading cause of death among pregnant women. Use of seat belts is extremely important for pregnant women, but the belts should be applied correctly. The lap belt must be worn low (below the uterus) and pulled tight across the pelvis (not abdomen). The shoulder belt is worn as usual. Proper use of belts helps prevent blunt injury to the uterus and fetus as well as protecting the mother.

Anatomy and Physiology

The unborn developing baby is called the fetus. The uterus or womb is a muscular sack in which the fetus develops. Since the blood of the mother and the fetus do not mix, there must be a way to provide food and oxygen and remove waste products from the fetus. The placenta is a vascular organ that attaches to the inside of the uterus. It functions as a membrane to allow oxygen and food to cross from mother's blood to baby's blood and for waste products to cross from baby's blood to mother's blood. The placenta is needed only during pregnancy, so it separates from the wall of the uterus at birth and is expelled after the birth of the baby. The placenta is thus often called the "afterbirth." If the placenta separates before birth (abruptio placentae), it can cause severe bleeding. The baby's blood is carried to and from the placenta through the umbilical cord. The umbilical cord is cut and tied off after birth since the placenta is no longer needed. While inside the uterus the fetus is completely enclosed within a thin membrane called the amniotic sac. This membrane also contains one or two pints of a liquid called amniotic fluid. The fetus floats in this "bag of waters" until just before birth, when the amniotic sac breaks and the fluid gushes out of the vagina or birth canal. This often signals the beginning of the birth process or labor. The opening of the uterus is the cervix. It is closed during pregnancy but must open or dilate to about 10 centimeters (4 inches) during the birth process to allow the baby to pass out of the uterus and into the birth canal.

Changes during Pregnancy

During the first 3 months of pregnancy, the fetus is being formed. The fetus remains quite small, so there is little growth of the uterus during this period. After the third month, the uterus grows rapidly, reaching the umbilicus by the fifth month and the epigastrium by the seventh month.

There are many other changes in the woman's body during this time. The blood volume, cardiac output, and heart rate are increased while the blood pressure is usually decreased slightly and there is slowed peristalsis in the gastro-intestinal tract. One very important change is the massive increase in the number and size of blood vessels around the uterus.

Figure 12–1. Anatomy of pregnancy. Uterus at 3 months and 8 months.

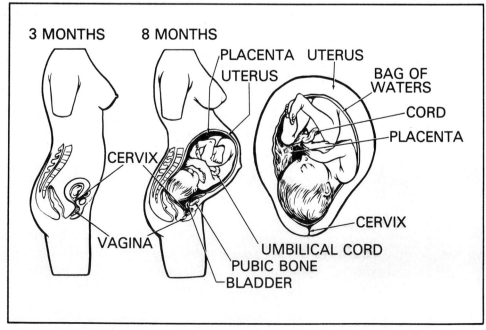

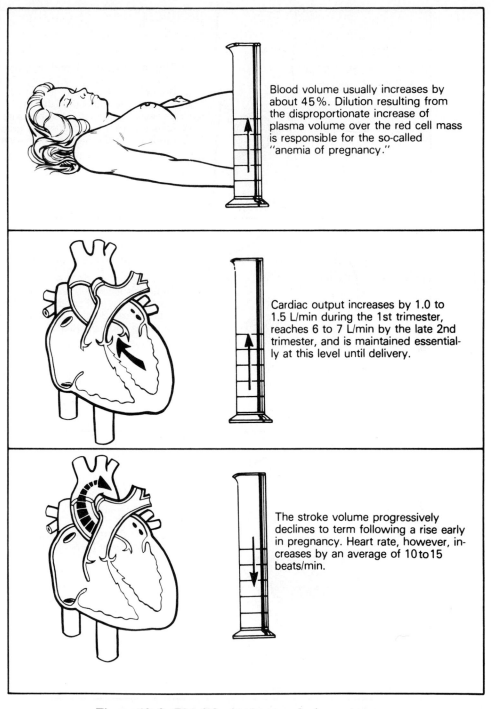

Blood volume usually increases by about 45%. Dilution resulting from the disproportionate increase of plasma volume over the red cell mass is responsible for the so-called "anemia of pregnancy."

Cardiac output increases by 1.0 to 1.5 L/min during the 1st trimester, reaches 6 to 7 L/min by the late 2nd trimester, and is maintained essentially at this level until delivery.

The stroke volume progressively declines to term following a rise early in pregnancy. Heart rate, however, increases by an average of 10 to 15 beats/min.

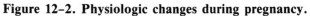

Figure 12-2. Physiologic changes during pregnancy.

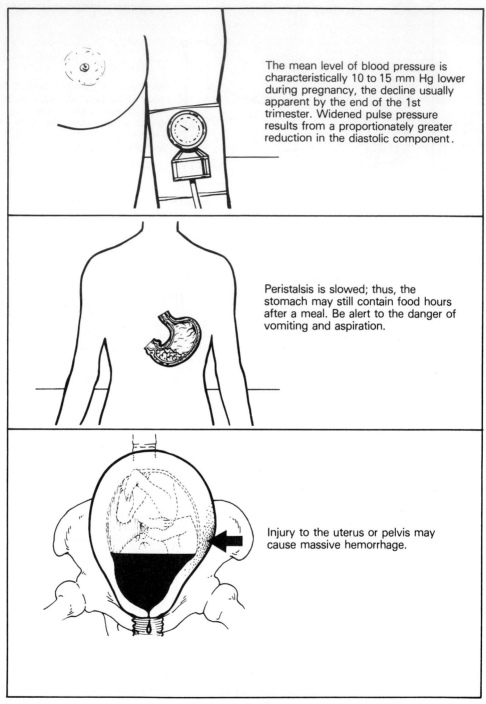

The mean level of blood pressure is characteristically 10 to 15 mm Hg lower during pregnancy, the decline usually apparent by the end of the 1st trimester. Widened pulse pressure results from a proportionately greater reduction in the diastolic component.

Peristalsis is slowed; thus, the stomach may still contain food hours after a meal. Be alert to the danger of vomiting and aspiration.

Injury to the uterus or pelvis may cause massive hemorrhage.

FIG. 12–2 (Cont.):

Types of Injuries

Obviously, the pregnant patient may sustain any injury that any other victim is subject to, but during the last 6 months of pregnancy, the large uterus and fetus are particularly subject to certain injuries. Injuries to the uterus may be blunt or penetrating. In both cases the greatest danger to mother and baby is hemorrhage and hemorrhagic shock.

A. *Penetrating injuries:* These are usually caused by gunshot or stab wounds. Since the uterus is anterior and usually quite large, it is frequently struck by penetrating objects. There are many very large blood vessels associated with the pregnant uterus, so massive hemorrhage may occur.

B. *Blunt trauma:* The most common cause of this is automobile accident injuries, but falls or beatings also can cause injury. The uterus is well designed to protect the baby. The fetus is inside the body, inside a muscular chamber that is filled with fluid; these elements work together to provide a very efficient "shock absorber" so that most minor trauma to the abdomen, such a blow or fall, does not harm the fetus. An automobile accident is a different story; the magnitude of force here is often great. The uterus, because of its size and location, is frequently injured. Sudden, blunt trauma to the abdomen during the later months of pregnancy may cause uterine rupture, abruptio placentae (premature separation of the placenta from the uterine wall), premature labor, or severe bleeding from injury to the large vessels. Usual abdominal blunt trauma injuries, such as ruptured spleen or liver, may also occur. There is a good chance that rupture of the diaphragm will occur with blunt trauma during later pregnancy. Multiple trauma with fracture of the pelvis can cause laceration or tearing of the vessels in the pelvis with massive hemorrhage. The common problem with almost all of the blunt injuries to the pregnant abdomen or pelvis is massive bleeding and hemorrhagic shock.

Evaluation of the Pregnant Trauma Victim

The priorities are the same.

1. Secure the airway and stabilize the spine.
2. Assess breathing and circulation.
3. Stop significant bleeding.

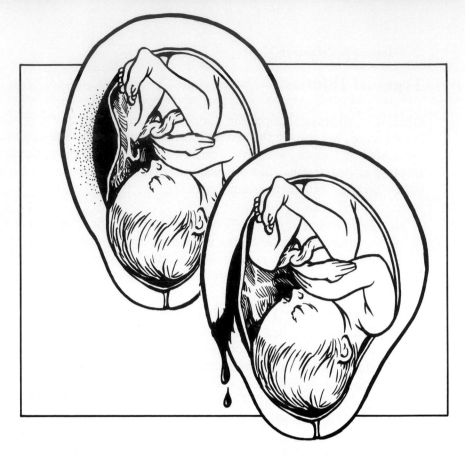

Figure 12–3. Blunt trauma to uterus. Blunt trauma may cause separation of the placenta or rupture of the uterus. Massive bleeding may occur.

4. Make a decision about critical trauma situations. If a critical situation is present, transfer the patient to a backboard and transport immediately. If no critical situation is apparent, transfer the patient to a backboard and proceed to the secondary survey.
5. Perform secondary survey, including neurological examination and splinting fractures.
6. Transport with continuous monitoring.

The things to remember are these:

1. The pregnant woman has a pulse rate that is 10 to 15 beats per minute faster than normal, and the blood pressure is lower than normal (but with widened rather than narrowed pulse pressure), so you may mistake the vital signs as being suggestive of shock when they are normal for the pregnant state.

158

2. The woman in later pregnancy may have a blood volume that is 20 to 45 percent higher than normal. This means that she might lose much more blood internally before symptoms of shock occur.

3. Because of the confusing vital signs in pregnancy and the extra blood volume, you must be alert or you will be late in diagnosing the development of hemorrhagic shock.

4. Trauma to the abdomen may cause bleeding inside the uterus. Mark the top of the uterus with a marking pencil. Enlargement of the uterus suggests intrauterine bleeding.

5. Monitor vital signs frequently and watch the abdomen for signs of intra-abdominal bleeding.

Management of the Pregnant Trauma Victim

Management of most injuries is the same as for those previously discussed, but there are certain things that are done differently.

A. *Volume replacement:* Hemorrhagic shock is the greatest danger from injuries to the uterus. The antishock garment can be used, but inflate only the legs; inflation of the abdominal compartment cuts off blood flow to the baby.

B. *Oxygen administration:* The oxygen requirement of the woman in later pregnancy is 10 to 20 percent greater than normal. There are two lives that depend on adequate oxygenation. As a general rule, all injured pregnant women are given oxygen.

C. *Vomiting:* Because of slow peristalsis and slow emptying of the stomach, there is a greater chance of the patient vomiting and choking. Be ready.

D. *Transport:* If you transport a woman in later pregnancy on her back, the uterus will press on the inferior vena cava, obstructing the flow of blood back to the heart. This can cause a 30 percent decrease in cardiac output, which in many cases is enough to cause shock and loss of blood flow to the baby. After the first 3 to 4 months of pregnancy, never transport the woman flat on her back. If there is no danger of spinal injury, you should transport her on her left side. If there is danger of spinal injury, you may secure her to a long spine board, but prop the board up slightly on the right side so that the uterus is leaning to the left side; this prevents compression of the vena cava (which runs on the right side). Be careful not to tip her over onto the floor; pregnant patients are top heavy. If the mother dies during

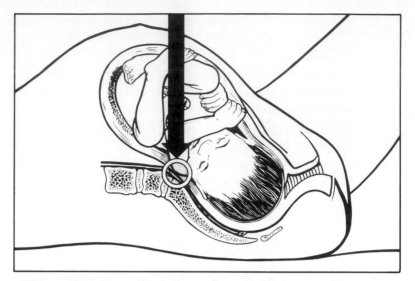

Figure 12–4. Venous return to the heart may be greatly compromised by uterine compression. Transport victim on her left side or tilt spine board to the left.

the prehospital phase, the fetus may still survive. You should transport rapidly while providing CPR and hyperventilation with high-flow oxygen. Notify medical control so that the hospital is prepared to do immediate cesarean section if the fetus is alive when you arrive.

Important Points to Remember

1. The most common cause of traumatic fetal death is death of the mother, so the goal of prehospital care is to get the mother to the emergency room alive. This gives both the mother and the fetus the best chance for survival.

2. Shock is more difficult to diagnose in the pregnant patient but is the most likely cause of prehospital death from injury to the uterus. Shock also kills the baby quickly since the blood supply to the fetus is shut off when the mother is in shock.

3. If there is any chance of hypoxia, give oxygen.

4. Transport the patient on her left side or tilt the backboard so that she is leaning to the left; this prevents obstruction of the vena cava and makes aspiration less likely if she vomits.

Chapter 13

PEDIATRIC TRAUMA

Trauma is the number one killer of children. After the newborn period, 50 percent of childhood deaths are due to trauma. As stated earlier, the general priorities are the same for children as for adults, but children are not simply "little adults." You must keep in mind the differences when evaluating and treating the injured infant or child. To appreciate the abnormal you must learn the normal. Since children come in all sizes, you must remember some generalizations about various age groups.

Respiratory Rate

Respiratory rate is influenced by many factors, such as fear, shock, drugs, or head injury. Although important, it is not as useful as some of the other signs. Normal respiratory rates are as follows:

1. *Infant:* 40 to 60 per minute
2. *Young child:* 20 to 30 per minute
3. *Older child:* 12 to 20 per minute

Blood pressure

The blood pressure is difficult to obtain in a small child. You must have a cuff that has a width of about three-fourths of the width of the child's upper arm in order to obtain an accurate blood pressure. You may even need a Doppler to hear accurate blood pressure. However, most ambulances are not equipped to obtain accurate blood pressure readings in small children. You must therefore learn to diagnose shock by observation of other signs.

Hypotensive Values

1. *Neonate:* less than 50 mmHg
2. *Infant:* less than 60 mmHg
3. *Child (up to 6):* less than 70 mmHg
4. *Child (older than 6):* less than 90 mmHg

Heart Rate

Although easily measured, this value is often influenced by fright (catecholamine release). Repeated determinations are important.

Table 13–1

TACHYCARDIA VALUES IN CHILDREN
Newborn over 200
infant over 180
child over 150
adolescent over 120

Airway and Ventilation

The small child has a large head and a short neck. His mandible is relatively small and his tongue relatively large. This makes mouth breathing difficult. Up to about the age of 6 months, infants can breathe through their mouths only when they are crying.

Diagnosis of Airway Obstruction

Observation is very important in diagnosing both the type and cause of airway obstruction. You should note the rate and depth of respiration. Look for nasal flaring and intercostal as well as sternal and supraclavicular retractions. Listen for wheezing, grunting, snoring, or stridor. Notice whether the ribs are used in respiration or whether there is diaphragmatic breathing only. Notice skin color and sensorium; the hypoxic child will be cyanotic or pale and either agitated (early hypoxia or fear) or lethargic (late hypoxia).

Normal respiration is not audible. When you hear abnormal breath sounds, you should think of airway obstruction. Wheezing is most commonly heard during expiration. It may be from bronchospasm (asthma), but it may also be from airway obstruction due to other causes, such as edema (swelling) or foreign body aspiration. Grunting with expiration is heard most commonly in infants with partial airway obstruction. It should be noted with alarm, for complete airway obstruction can follow. Snoring is caused by oropharyngeal or nasopharyngeal partial obstruction. It is most commonly caused by the tongue falling back into the posterior pharynx in the unconscious victim. Stridor is usually harsh and high pitched. It is most commonly heard on inhalation. Stridor is a sign of tight upper airway obstruction, such as laryngeal edema.

Injuries to the airways are not common during infancy and childhood, but those seen most often in the prehospital environment are the following:

1. *Foreign body aspiration:* Half of all cases are caused by peanuts. Small children tend to examine new things by putting them in their mouths.

Figure 13–1. Signs of respiratory distress.

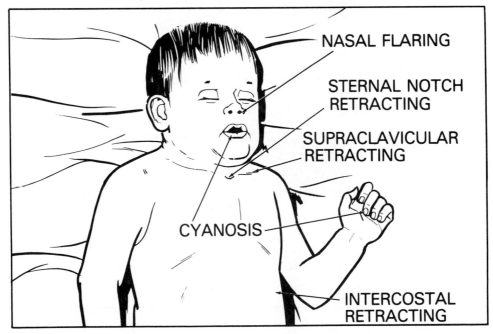

You should always have a high index of suspicion of foreign body aspiration in children who suddenly develop airway difficulty.

2. *Impact injuries to the face or neck:* These may cause airway obstruction from edema or from actual laryngotracheal disruption. There can be compression of the airways and severe respiratory distress with only minimal external signs of soft tissue injury to the neck.

3. *Chemical or thermal burns:* The upper airways are so small in children that even minimal swelling can cause major airway obstructions.

In general, mouth-to-mouth ventilation is best for children. You can stabilize the head and neck, open the airway with a jaw thrust, and give good ventilations without the assistance of another rescuer. Using a bag–valve mask requires two rescuers to maintain head and neck stability as well as good face seal and ventilations. It is difficult to judge airway compliance using the bag–valve mask. You are more likely to hypoventilate since airway resistance may be many times higher in a child than in an adult. Bag–valve masks, if used, should not have a pop-off valve. Keep suction available since vomiting and aspiration are much more common in children than in adults.

Figure 13–2. Mouth-to-mouth ventilation in a child.

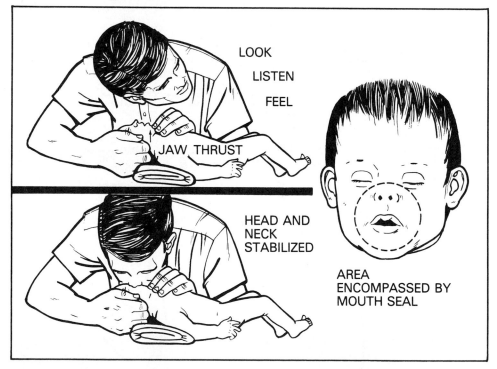

Chest Trauma

An important difference (from adults) is that children's ribs are so flexible that flail chest is uncommon. Pulmonary contusions and diaphragmatic hernias are more common because children are more commonly run over by wheels. Be very alert for development of tension pneumothorax.

Shock

Circulating blood volume is only 7 to 8 percent of body weight, so a small blood loss in a child may be sufficient to cause hemorrhagic shock. A 1-year-old child (10 kg) with a 2-inch laceration will bleed just as much as an adult (70 kg) with the same laceration. The adult has 5000 cc of circulating blood volume, whereas the child has only 750 cc. If each bled 200 cc from his wound, the adult would have no ill effects, but the child would be in obvious hemorrhagic shock. The diagnosis of shock in a child requires careful observation. The most important signs are the following:

1. Pallor (secondary to decreased skin perfusion)
2. Altered sensorium (secondary to decreased brain perfusion)

Blood pressure is difficult to determine accurately in the small child, so is of little use in the diagnosis of shock. It is common for the traumatized child to become hypovolemic due to shock from bleeding into the chest or abdomen with no external blood loss. The child in shock should be rapidly transported to the hospital. You should load the victim and transport. Often a car may be quite adequate if an ambulance is not available. In a small child the extremities can be wrapped with elastic bandages to achieve the same results as antishock trousers. A larger child may have the pediatric antishock garment applied. These may be applied in the transport vehicle. Do not waste the golden hour.

All children in shock should receive 100 percent oxygen if possible.

All children in shock should be wrapped to prevent hypothermia.

Spinal Cord Trauma

The same principles apply for children as for adults. Spinal cord injury is less common in children but does occur. Children should always have their spines stabilized.

Head Trauma

Head trauma is the major cause of death from trauma in children. However, children with severe head injuries have a better chance of surviving with a good neurological recovery than do adults with the same types of injuries. Adults with decerebrate posturing have a grim prognosis, but over 89 percent of children with decerebrate posturing will survive. Most children with a Glascow Coma Scale of 5 to 7 will live with a good functional recovery. Only 50 percent of adults will do well. The point here is that you must be aggressive in trying to save the child with what appears to be a severe head injury.

The most common pathological finding for children who die of brain injury is a diffuse swelling of the brain. This swelling seems to be from an increase in cerebral blood volume and not from edema fluid. In children the initial response of the injured brain is vasodilitation with increased cerebral blood flow and increased cerebral blood volume. This causes increased intracranial pressure, which causes pressure on brain structures. This, in turn, causes coma, respiratory arrest, and finally death.

Survival of children with head injuries depends on lowering intracranial pressure. Since this pressure is caused by increased cerebral blood volume, the treatment is to constrict the cerebral vessels. This decreases the accumulation of blood in the injured areas of the brain and prevents dangerous rises in intracerebral pressure.

Hyperventilation is the best method for achieving cerebral vasoconstriction. You can begin hyperventilation in the field. This removes carbon dioxide from the body and within minutes the intracerebral pressure will decrease. Hyperventilation will remove enough carbon dioxide to cause a 50 percent constriction in cerebral blood vessels. This early lowering of intracerebral pressure is a critical part of the therapy of head injuries. If a child with a possible head injury begins to develop altered consciousness, you should immediately begin hyperventilation with 100 percent oxygen.

Remember that spinal cord injuries are more common in head injury victims. Usually, a victim with even a severe head injury will have some motion of his extremities. If the arms and legs are flaccid, you should expect spinal cord injury.

Extremity Trauma

The principles are the same as for adults. Small children usually do not require traction splints for leg fractures.

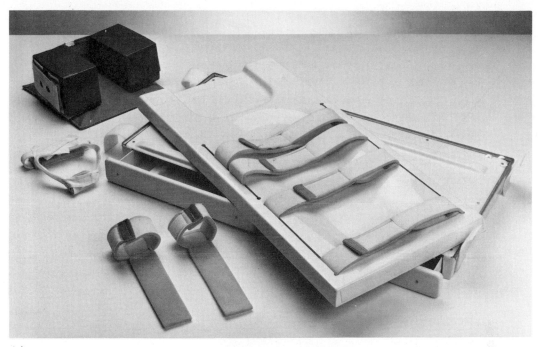

(a)

Figure 13-3a. Components of
the Clark Pediatric Unit[R].
Figure 13-3b. Example of an
infant immobilized on a Clark
Pediatric Unit[R].

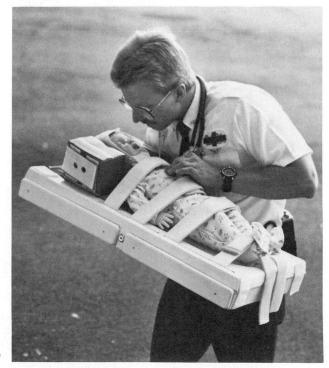

(b)

Abdominal Trauma

Blunt trauma is most common in small children. Liver injury is more common in children because the liver is relatively larger than in adults. Liver injuries are second only to head injuries as the major cause of traumatic death in children. Be very suspicious for abdominal injury in children. Any abdominal tenderness should alert you to be prepared for the development of hemorrhagic shock.

Burns

The principles are the same as for adults. Be aware especially of inhalation injuries, since even slight swelling can cause airway obstruction in children.

General Approach to the Injured Child

The priorities are the same as for adults:

1. Airway maintenance and control of cervical spine.
2. Assessment of breathing and circulation.
3. Control of bleeding.
4. Decision about critical trauma situations. If a critical situation is present, transfer the child to a backboard and transport immediately. If no critical situation is apparent, transfer the child to a backboard and proceed to the secondary survey.
5. Secondary survey and splinting of fractures.
6. Transport with continuous monitoring.

As a general rule, you should not separate the injured child from his parents. If the parent(s) and the child are both seriously injured, you may require two ambulances to care for each of them properly. Children are so portable that they can (and should) be transported rapidly. There are very few procedures that should be done in the field. An EMT first responder may package a child and transport by automobile before the ambulance arrives. One recent study found that most injured children, if transported by automobile, could have been in the emergency room before the ambulance arrived at the scene. Remember that children are often more frightened than adults (even more frightened than you are at having to treat them), so talk gently to them and handle them gently.

Chapter 14

CRITICAL TRAUMA SITUATIONS: "LOAD and GO"

There are certain situations that require hospital treatment within minutes if the victim is to have any chance for survival. The primary survey is designed to identify these situations. When these situations are recognized, the victim should be loaded immediately onto a backboard, transferred to the ambulance, and transported rapidly with lights and siren. Lifesaving procedures may be needed but should be done during transport. Nonlifesaving procedures (such as splinting and bandaging) must not hold up transport.

Critical Situations That Require "Load and Go"

1. Airway obstruction that cannot be quickly relieved by mechanical methods such as suction or forceps
2. Conditions resulting in possible inadequate breathing
   a. Large open chest wound (sucking chest wound)
   b. Large flail chest
   c. Tension pneumothorax
   d. Major blunt chest injury
3. Traumatic cardiopulmonary arrest
4. Shock
5. Head injury with unconsciousness, unequal pupils, or decreasing level of consciousness

Assessment findings that should alert you to possible critical trauma conditions are as follows:

1. Cervical spine control with evaluation of Airway and initial level of consciousness

Critical Findings	*Possible Causes*
a. Unresponsive or poorly responsive	Head injury, cardiac arrest, or late shock
b. No movement of air	Airway obstruction or cardio-respiratory arrest
c. Respiratory difficulty	Airway obstruction or chest injury

2. Assess Breathing and Circulation.

Critical Findings	*Possible Causes*
a. No respiration	Cardiac arrest
b. Difficulty with rate or depth of respiration	Slow or irregular—head injury Fast, shallow—shock or chest injury
c. No pulse	Cardiac arrest Late shock
d. Pulse at neck but not at wrist	Late shock
e. Slow capillary refill	Early shock
f. Rapid, weak pulse (>100 per minute)	Shock

3. Examine the neck.

Critical Findings	*Possible Causes*
a. Discoloration and swelling	Developing airway obstruction
b. Distended neck veins and/or deviated trachea, respiratory difficulty, shock	Tension pneumothorax
c. Distended neck veins and shock	Pericardial tamponade

4. Examine the chest.

Critical Findings	*Possible Causes*
a. Sucking chest wound	Open pneumothorax
b. Hyperresonant on one side, respiratory difficulty, shock, distended neck veins	Tension pneumothorax

c. Unstable segment of chest wall or sternum, difficulty breathing	Flail chest
d. Difficulty breathing, breath sounds decreased on one side, crepitation	Major thoracic airway injury
e. Contusion or puncture wound of anterior chest, shock, distended neck veins	Cardiac tamponade Myocardial contusion
f. Penetrating chest wound, shock	Hemothorax Heart wound Major thoracic vascular injury

5. Control active bleeding.

Critical Findings	*Possible Cause*
Major blood loss or poorly controlled bleeding	Major vascular injury

At this point you should be able to make a decision about critical trauma conditions and who should be in the "load and go" category. Any victim with these symptoms falls in the "load and go" category:

1. Shock
2. Respiratory difficulty
3. Decreased level of consciousness

Any victim with injuries that will rapidly lead to shock or respiratory difficulty should be in the "load and go" category. This includes large flail chest or open pneumothorax even though they may not demonstrate respiratory difficulty at the time of the primary survey. The same is true of massive or poorly controlled bleeding even if shock is not evident at the time of the primary survey.

Secondary Survey

If the victim does not appear to have a critical trauma situation, you may perform the secondary survey before transport. During the secondary survey there are a few conditions that will change the victim's category to "load and go." Be very suspicious of those patients in whom the mechanisms of injury are such that severe injuries could have occurred. Such patients may suddenly deteriorate.

1. Development of shock, respiratory difficulty, or decreasing level of consciousness
2. The finding of a tender, distended abdomen
3. Bilateral femur fractures
4. Unstable pelvis

Findings 2, 3, and 4 so commonly lead to shock that these victims should be taken to the emergency department without delay. In all "load and go" situations you should call ahead to have the emergency department and possibly the operating room prepared for your arrival. If a specific surgeon is needed, your medical control physician can have him called before you arrive. Rapid transport is not lifesaving if the necessary surgeon is not available to treat the victim when he arrives. The true test of an EMS system is whether every phase of emergency care can work together as a team when a life depends on definitive care within a matter of minutes.

Skill Station 1

UPPER AIRWAY MANAGEMENT

Objectives

The objectives of this skill station are as follows:

1. To learn the various manual methods of opening the airway.
2. To learn how to suction the airway.
3. To learn how to insert a nasopharyngeal and oropharyngeal airway.
4. To learn how to use the pocket mask.
5. To learn how to use the bag–valve mask.

Procedures

   I. Manual techniques to open the airway
      A. Modified jaw thrust
         1. Place your hands on either side of the neck at the base of the skull.
         2. While maintaining in-line stabilization of the neck, push up on the angles of the mandible with your thumbs.

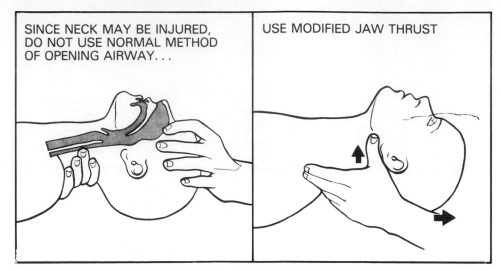

SINCE NECK MAY BE INJURED, DO NOT USE NORMAL METHOD OF OPENING AIRWAY...

USE MODIFIED JAW THRUST

Figure S1–1. Modified jaw thrust.

B. *Jaw thrust*
1. Stabilize the head and neck with your knees or have your partner stabilize the neck in a neutral position.
2. Using the index and middle fingers of each hand, grasp the angles of the jaw just below the ears.
3. Lift gently.
C. *Chin lift*
1. Stabilize the head and neck with your knees or have your partner stabilize the neck in a neutral position.
2. Place the fingers of one hand under the chin.
3. With the thumb of the same hand, grasp the chin below the lower lip.
4. Lift gently.
D. *Jaw lift* (used for inserting oral airway or esophageal airway)
1. Stabilize the head and neck with your knees or have your partner stabilize the neck in a neutral position.
2. Place the fingers of one hand under the chin.
3. Insert the thumb of the same hand inside the mouth. Grasp the lower incisors.
4. Lift gently.

II. Suctioning the airway
A. Attach the suction tubing to the portable suction machine.
B. Turn the device on and test it.

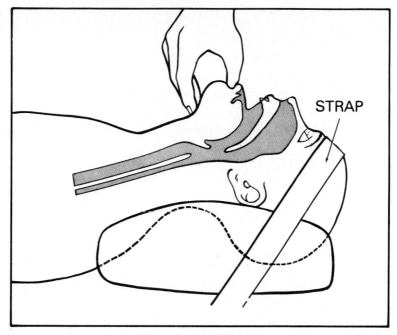

Figure S1–2. Chin lift.

Figure S1–3. Jaw lift.

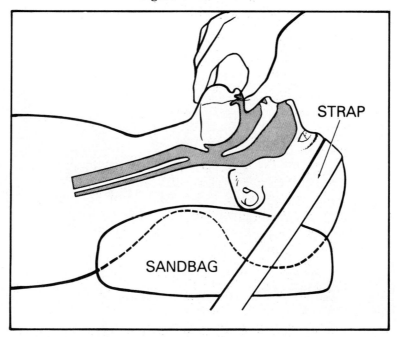

    C.   Insert the suction tube through the nose or mouth without activating the suction.

    D.   Activate the suction and withdraw the suction tube.

    E.   Repeat the procedure as necessary.

III. Insertion of pharyngeal airways

    A. Nasopharyngeal airway

        1.   Choose the appropriate size. It should be the largest that will fit easily through the external nares.

        2.   Lubricate the tube.

        3.   Insert it straight back through the right nostril with the beveled edge of the airway toward the septum.

        4.   To insert it in the left nostril, turn the airway upside down so that the bevel is toward the septum, then insert straight back through the nostril until you reach the posterior pharynx. At this point, turn the airway over 180 degrees and insert it down the pharynx until it lies behind the tongue.

Figure S1–4. Insertion of nasopharyngeal airway into right nostril.

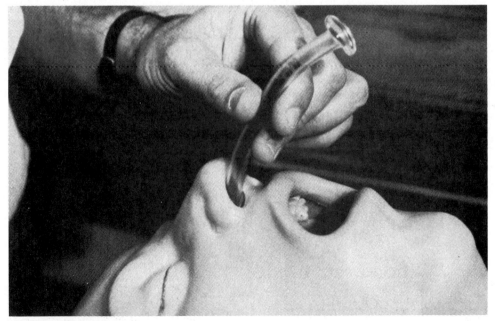

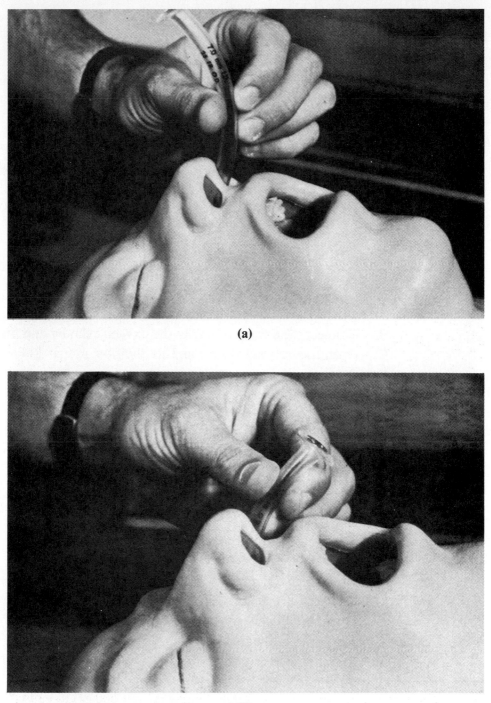

(a)

(b)

Figure S1–5a. Insertion of nasopharyngeal airway into left
nostril. Insert upside down so bevel is toward the septum.
Figure S1–5b. When tip is to the back of the pharynx, rotate
airway 180 degrees.

    B.   *Oropharyngeal airway*
1. Choose the appropriate size
2. Open the airway.
   a. Scissor maneuver
   b. Jaw lift
   c. Tongue blade
3. Insert the airway gently without pushing the tongue back into the pharynx.
   a. Insert the airway upside down and rotate into place. This method should not be used in children.
   b. Insert the airway under direct vision using the tongue blade.

IV. **Use of pocket mask with supplemental oxygen**

    A.   Have your partner stabilize the neck in a neutral position (or apply a good stabilization device).

    B.   Connect the oxygen tubing to the oxygen cylinder and the mask.

    C.   Open the oxygen cylinder and set the flow rate at 12 liters/min.

    D.   Open the airway.

    E.   Insert the oral airway properly.

    F.   Place the mask on the face and establish a good seal.

    G.   Ventilate mouth to mask with enough volume (about 800 to 1000 cc) to cause the green light to come on in the recording mannequin.

V. **Use of the bag–valve mask**

    A.   Stabilize the neck with a suitable device.

    B.   Connect the oxygen tubing to the bag–valve system and oxygen cylinder.

    C.   Attach the oxygen reservoir to the bag–valve mask.

    D.   Open the oxygen cylinder and set the flow rate at 12 liters/min.

    E.   Select the proper size mask and attach it to the bag–valve device.

    F.   Open the airway.

    G.   Insert the oral airway properly.

    H.   Place the mask on the face and have your partner establish and maintain a good seal.

    I.   Ventilate with enough volume (about 800 cc) to cause the green light to come on in the recording mannequin. Use both hands.

    J.   If you are forced to ventilate without a partner, use one hand to maintain a face seal and the other to squeeze the bag. This

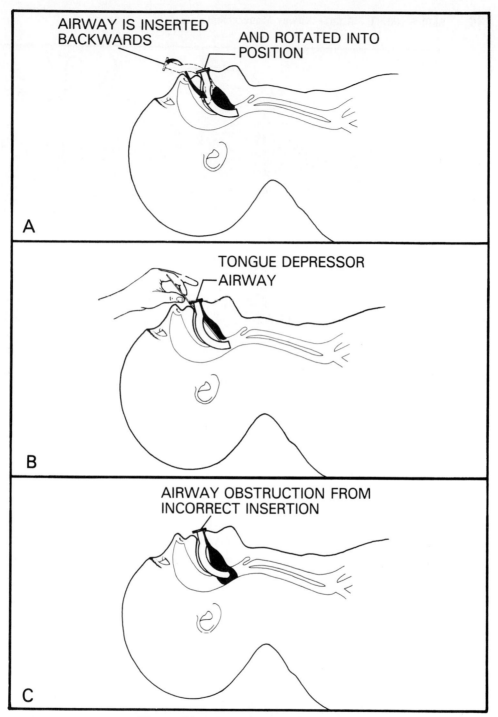

Figure S1–6. Insertion of oral airway.

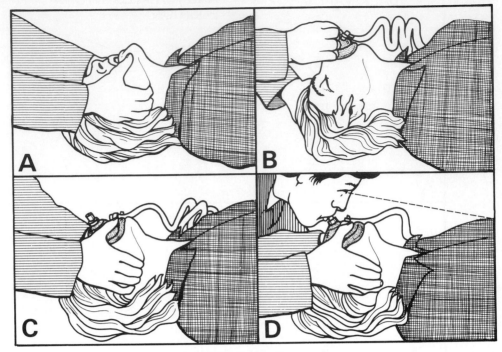

Figure S1–7. Pocket mask.

decreases the volume of ventilation because less volume is produced by only one hand squeezing the bag.

K.   Hyperventilate. All trauma victims who have decreased level of consciousness should be hyperventilated with 100 percent oxygen at a rate of one ventilation about every 2 seconds (24 to 30 breaths per minute). Using procedure steps A to I above, practice hyperventilation until you feel comfortable with the rhythm of ventilating at the rate of 24 to 30 breaths per minute.

Skill Station 2

A. SPINAL IMMOBILIZATION— SHORT BACKBOARD

Objectives

The objectives of this skill station are as follows:

1. To learn when to use spinal immobilization.
2. To learn the correct technique of spinal immobilization with a short backboard.

I. Who should have spinal immobilization?

A. Any victim of trauma with obvious neurological deficit such as paralysis, weakness, or paresthesia (numbness or tingling)

B. Any victim of trauma who complains of pain in the head, neck, or back

C. Any victim of trauma who is unconscious

D. Any victim of trauma who may have injury to the spine but in whom evaluation is difficult due to altered mental status (e.g., drugs, alcohol)

E. Any unconscious patient who may have been subjected to trauma

    F.   Any trauma victim with facial or head injuries

    G.   Any trauma victim subjected to deceleration forces

    H.   When in doubt, immobilize

  II. **When to immobilize**

Patients requiring immobilization must have it done before they are moved at all. In the case of an automobile accident, the victim must be immobilized before he is removed from the wreckage. More movement is involved in extrication than at any other time, so immobilization of neck and spine must be accomplished before beginning extrication.

  III. **Technique of spinal immobilization using the short backboard**

This device is for use in the patient who is in a position (such as an automobile) that does not allow use of the long backboard. There are several different devices of this type; some devices have different strapping mechanisms from the one explained here. You must become familiar with the equipment you will employ before using it in the field.

    A.   Remember that the routine priorities of evaluation and management are done before the immobilization devices go on.

    B.   One EMT must, if possible, station himself behind the victim, place his hands on either side of the victim's head, and immobilize the neck in a neutral position. This step is part of the ABCs of evaluation. It is done at the same time that you begin evaluation of the airway.

    C.   When you have the patient stable enough to begin splinting, you must apply a rigid extrication collar. If you have enough people, this can be done while someone else is doing the ABCs of evaluation and management.

    D.   Position the backboard behind the victim. The first EMT continues to immobilize the neck while the short backboard is being maneuvered into place. The victim may have to be moved forward to get the backboard in place; great care must be taken that moves are coordinated so as to support the neck and back.

    E.   Secure the victim to the board: there are usually two straps for this. Bring each strap over a leg, down between both legs, back around the outside of the same leg, and then across the chest, then attach them to the opposite upper straps that were brought across the shoulders.

    F.   Tighten the straps until the victim is held securely.

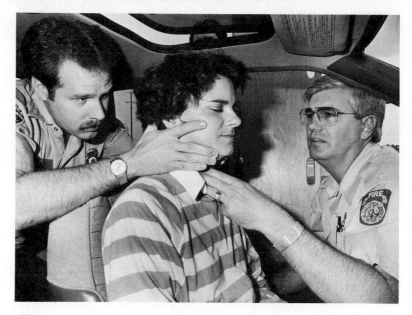

Figure S2–1. Stabilize the neck and perform the primary survey.

Figure S2–2. Apply a rigid extrication collar.

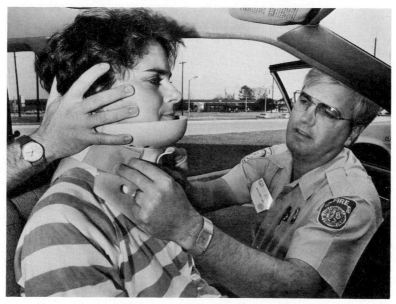

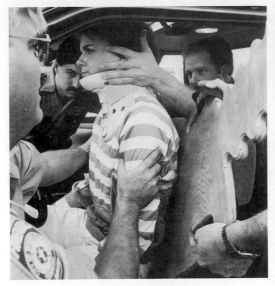

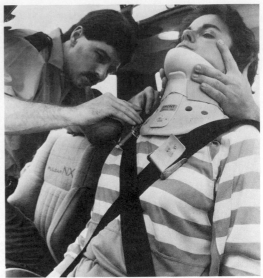

Figure S2–3. Position the short backboard behind the victim. Coordinate all movement so that the spine is kept immobile.

Figure S2–4. Apply straps and tighten securely.

G. Secure the victim's head to the board by wide tape or elastic wraps around the forehead. Apply padding under the neck and head as needed to maintain a neutral position.

H. Transfer the victim to a long backboard. Turn the victim so that his back is to the opening through which he is to be removed. Someone must support his legs so that the upper legs remain at a 90-degree angle to the torso. Position the long backboard through the opening until it is under the victim. Lower the victim back onto the long backboard and slide the victim and the short backboard up into position on the long backboard. Loosen the straps on the short board and allow the patient's legs to extend out flat and then retighten the straps. Now secure him to the long board with straps, and secure his head with a padded immobilization device. When he is secured in this way, it is possible to turn the whole board up on its side if the victim has to vomit. The patient should remain securely immobilized.

Important Points to Remember

1. When you are placing the straps around the legs on a male, do not catch the genitals in the straps.

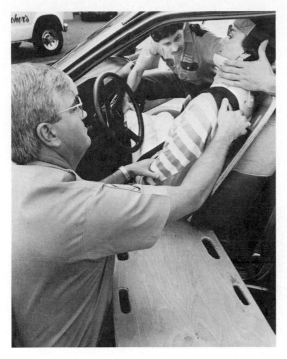

Figure S2–5. Turn the victim carefully then lower onto the long backboard.

Figure S2–6. Slide the victim and the short backboard up into position on the long backboard. Loosen the straps and allow the legs to extend out flat then retighten the straps. Secure the victim and the short backboard to the long backboard. Apply padded immobilization device to secure the victim's head and neck.

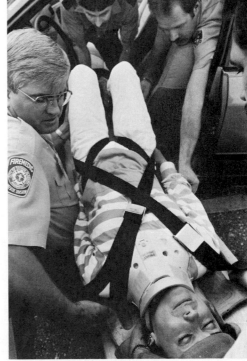

2. Do not use the short board as a "handle" to move the victim. Move both victim and board as a unit.

3. When you are applying the horizontal strap (long backboard) around a woman, place the upper strap above her breasts, not across them.

4. When you are applying the lower horizontal strap on a pregnant woman, see that it is low enough so as not to injure the fetus.

5. Injuries may force you to modify how you attach the straps.

6. The victim must be secured well enough to have no motion of the spine if the board is turned on its side.

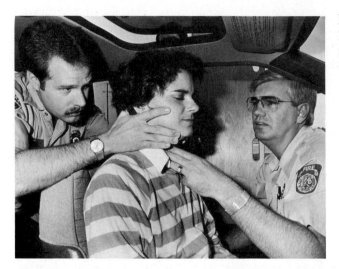

Figure S2–7. Kendrick Extrication Device (K.E.D.) Stabilize the neck and perform the primary survey.

Figure S2–8. Apply a rigid extrication collar.

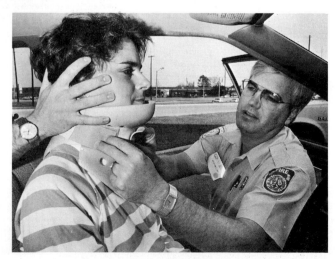

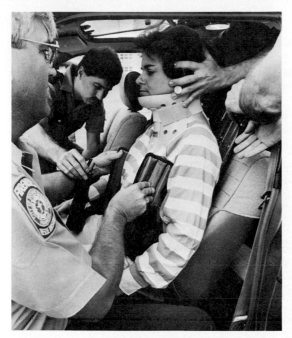

Figure S2-9. Position the device behind the victim. Coordinate all movements so that the spine is kept immobile. Position the chest panels up well into the armpits.

Figure S2-11. Loop each leg strap around the ipsilateral (same side) leg and back to the buckle on the same side. Fasten snugly.

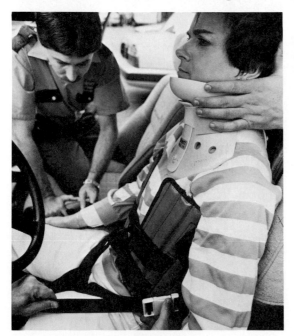

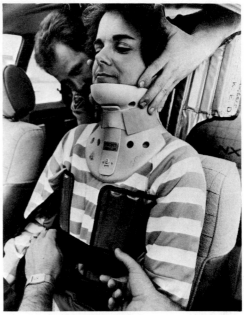

Figure S2-10. Tighten the chest straps.

187

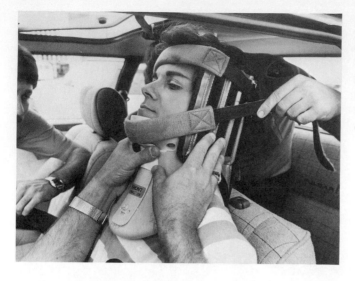

Figure S2–12. Apply firm padding as needed between the head and the headpiece to keep the head in a neutral position. Bring the head flaps around to the side of the head and secure firmly with straps, tape, or elastic wrap.

Figure S2–13. Turn the patient and the device as a unit, then lower onto a long backboard. Slide the patient and the device up into position on the board. Loosen the leg straps and allow the legs to extend out flat, then retighten the straps. Secure the patient and the device to the backboard.

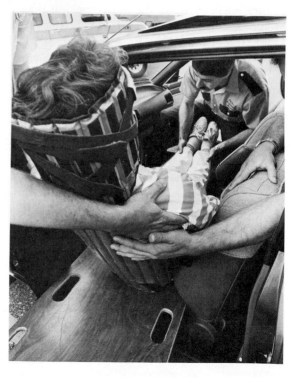

Skill Station 3

EMERGENCY RAPID EXTRICATION

Objective

The objective of this skill station is to learn indications and techniques of emergency rapid extrication.

Victims left inside vehicles after an accident are usually stabilized on a short backboard (or extrication device) and then transferred onto a long backboard. Although this is the best way to extricate anyone with a possible spinal injury, there are certain situations where a more rapid method must be used.

I. **Situations requiring emergency rapid extrication**
   A. Scene survey identifies a condition that may *immediately* endanger the victim (and the EMTs). *Examples:*
      1. Fire or immediate danger of fire
      2. Danger of explosion
      3. Rapidly rising water
      4. Structure in danger of collapse
   B. Primary survey of the victim identifies a condition that requires immediate intervention that cannot be done in the vehicle.

Examples:

1. Airway obstruction that is not relieved by jaw thrust or finger sweep
2. Cardiac or respiratory arrest
3. Chest or airway injuries requiring ventilation or assisted ventilation
4. Deep shock or bleeding that cannot be controlled

   This procedure is *only* to be used in a situation where the victim's life is in *immediate* danger. Whenever you use the procedure it should be noted in the run report and you should be prepared to defend your actions at a run review by your medical control physician. This is an example of "Desperate situations often demand desperate measures."

II. Procedure

A. One rescuer must, if possible, station himself behind the victim, place his hands on either side of the victim's head, and stabilize the neck in a neutral position. This step is part of the ABCs of evaluation. It is done at the same time that you begin evaluation of the airway.

B. Do a rapid survey as you quickly apply a cervical collar. You should have the collar with you when you begin.

Figure S3–1. Stabilize the neck and perform the primary survey.

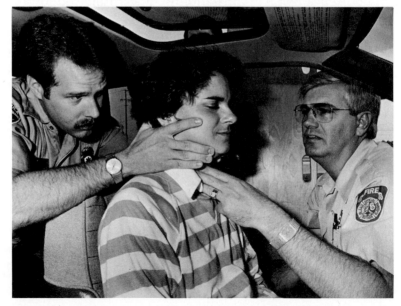

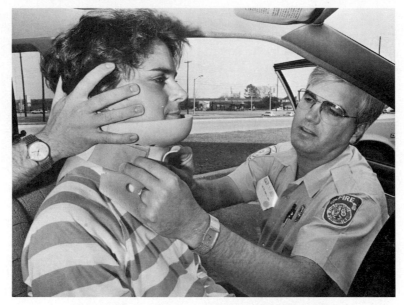

Figure S3-2. Apply a rigid extrication collar.

C. If your scene survey or your primary survey of the victim reveals an immediate life-threatening situation, go to the emergency rapid extrication technique described below. This requires at least four and preferably five or six persons to perform well.

D. Immediately slide the long backboard onto the seat and, if possible, at least slightly under the victim's buttocks.

E. A second EMT stands close beside the open door of the vehicle and takes over control of the cervical spine.

F. EMT number 1 or another EMT is positioned on the other side of the front seat ready to rotate the victim's legs around.

G. Another EMT is also positioned at the open door by the victim. By holding the upper torso, he works together with the EMT holding the legs to turn the victim carefully.

H. The victim is turned so that his back is toward the backboard. His legs are lifted and his back is lowered to the backboard. The neck and back are not allowed to bend during this maneuver.

I. Using teamwork, the victim is carefully slid to the full length of the backboard and his legs are carefully straightened.

J. The victim is then moved immediately away from the vehicle (to the ambulance if available) and resuscitation is begun. He is secured to the backboard as soon as possible.

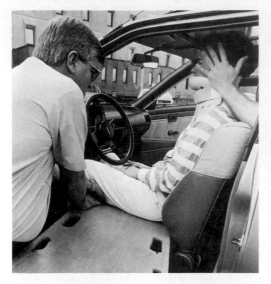

Figure S3–3. Slide the long backboard onto the seat and slightly under the patient.

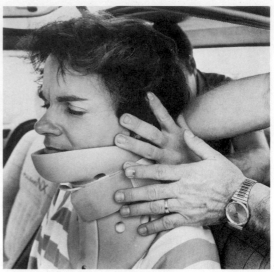

Figure S3–4. A second EMT stands close beside the open door of the vehicle and takes over control of the cervical spine.

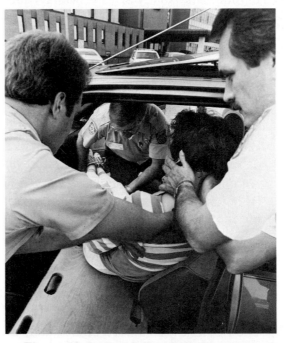

Figure S3–5. Carefully supporting the neck, torso, and legs, the EMTs turn the patient.

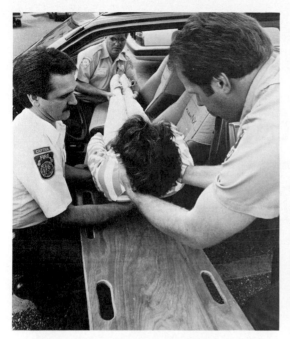

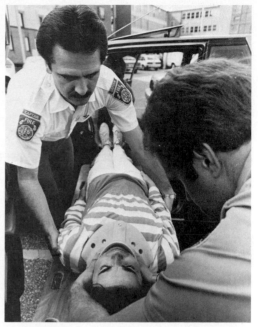

Figure S3–6. The legs are lifted and the back is lowered to the backboard.

Figure S3–7. Carefully slide the patient to the full length of the backboard.

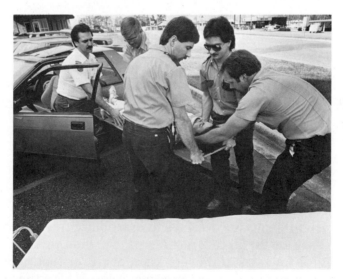

Figure S3–8. The patient is immediately moved away from the vehicle and into the ambulance, if available. Secure the patient to the backboard as soon as possible.

Skill Station 4

TRACTION SPLINTS

Objectives

The objectives of this skill station are as follows:

1. To learn when to use a traction splint
2. To learn the possible complications of using a traction splint
3. To learn how to apply the most common traction splints:
   a. Thomas splint.
   b. Hare splint.
   c. Klippel splint.
   d. Sager splint.
   e. Donway splint.

Traction splints are designed to immobilize fractures of the lower extremities. They are useful for fractures of the femur or upper tibia. They are not useful for fractures of the hip, knee, ankle, or foot. Applying firm traction to a fractured or dislocated knee may tear the blood vessels behind the knee. If there appears to be a pelvic fracture, you cannot use a traction splint because it may cause further damage to the pelvis. Fractures below the midthigh that are not angulated or severely shortened may just as well be immobilized by air splints or the antishock garment. Traction splints work by applying a padded device to the back of the pelvis (ischium) or to the groin. A hitching device is then applied to the ankle and countertraction is applied until the limb is straight and well immobilized. The splints must be applied to the pelvis and groin very carefully to prevent excessive pressure on the genitalia. Care must also be used when attaching the hitching device to the foot and ankle so as not to interfere with circulation. To prevent any unnecessary movement, traction splints should not be applied until the victim is on a long backboard. If the splint extends beyond the end of the backboard, you must be very careful when moving the victim and when closing the ambulance door. You must check the circulation in the injured leg, so remove the shoe before attaching the hitching device. In every case at least two EMTs are needed. One must hold steady, gentle traction on the foot and leg while the other applies the splint. When dealing with "load and go" situations the splint should not be applied until the victim is in the ambulance (unless the ambulance has not arrived).

A. *Thomas splint (half-ring splint)*
   1. The first EMT supports the leg and maintains gentle traction while the second EMT cuts away the clothing and removes the shoe and sock to check pulse and sensation at the foot.
   2. Position the splint under the injured leg. The ring goes down and the short side goes to the inside of the leg. Slide the ring snugly up under the hip, where it will be pressed against the ischial tuberosity.
   3. Position two support straps above the knee and two below the knee.
   4. Attach the top ring strap.
   5. Apply padding to the foot and ankle.
   6. Apply the traction hitch around the foot and ankle.
   7. Maintain gentle traction by hand.
   8. Attach the traction hitch to the end of the splint.
   9. Increase traction by Spanish windlass action using a stick or tongue depressors.
   10. Release manual traction and reassess ciculation and sensation.
   11. Support the end of the splint so that there is no pressure on the heel.

B. *Hare splint*
   1. Position the victim on the backboard or stretcher.
   2. The first EMT supports the leg and maintains gentle traction while the second EMT cuts away the clothing and removes the shoe and sock to check pulse and sensation at the foot.

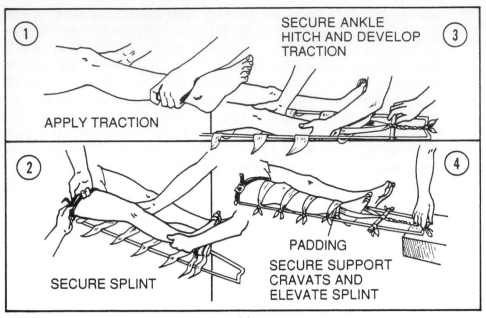

(a)

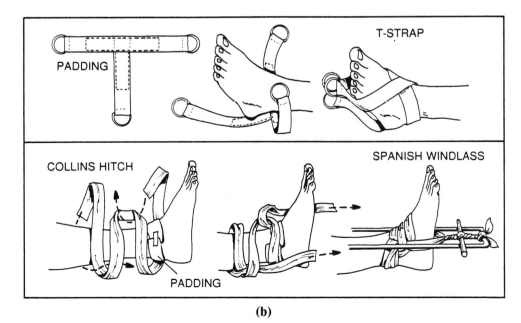

(b)

Figure S4–1A. Applying a traction (Thomas) splint.
Figure S4–1B. Applying a traction hitch to the ankle.

3. Position the splint under the injured leg. The ring goes down and the short side goes to the inside of the leg. Slide the ring up snugly under the hip against the ischial tuberosity.
4. Position two support straps above the knee and two below the knee.
5. Attach the heel rest.
6. Attach the top strap.
7. Apply the padded traction hitch to the ankle and foot.
8. Maintain gentle manual traction.
9. Attach the traction hitch to the windlass by way of the S-hook.
10. Turn the ratchet until the correct tension is applied.
11. Release manual traction and recheck circulation and sensation.
12. Attach support straps around the leg with Velcro straps.
13. To release traction, pull the ratchet knob outward and then slowly turn to loosen.

C. *Klippel splint*
1. Position the victim on the long backboard or stretcher.
2. The first EMT supports the leg and maintains gentle traction while the second EMT cuts away the clothing and removes the shoe and sock to check the pulse and sensation at the foot.
3. Using the uninjured leg as a guide, pull the splint out to the correct length.
4. Turn the footplate up by pushing to the side and then turning.
5. Turn the heel rest down by pushing in both knobs simultaneously and then turning.
6. While maintaining gentle traction and support, slide the splint under the leg (ring turned down) until the ring is snugly under the hip against the ischial tuberosity.
7. Position two support straps above the knee aand two below the knee.
8. Attach the top ring strap.
9. Push the footplate up against the sole of the foot. Push the two release levers to shorten the splint.
10. Apply padding to the foot and ankle.
11. Bring the traction hitch up under the ankle and then cross the two straps over the foot, around the footplate, and back over the foot, where they attach by Velcro fasteners.
12. While maintaining manual traction, extend the splint by pulling on the two rails until correct tension is obtained.
13. Release manual traction and recheck circulation and sensation.
14. Attach support straps around the leg with Velcro fasteners.

D. *Sager splint:* This splint is different in several ways. It works by providing countertraction against the pubic ramus and the ischial tuberosity medial to the shaft of the femur, thus does not go under the leg. The hip does not have to be slightly flexed as with the Hare and Klippel. The Sager is also lighter and more compact than other traction splints. You can also splint both legs with one splint if needed. The new Sagers are significantly improved over older models and may represent the "state of the art" in traction splints.

Figure S4–2A. Sager Traction Splint.
Figure S4–2B. Patient with both legs splinted with Sager Traction Splint.

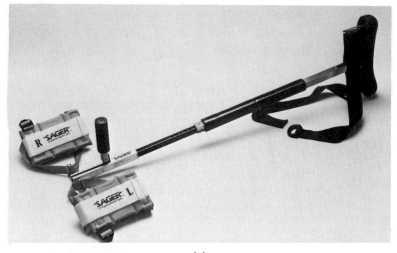

(a)

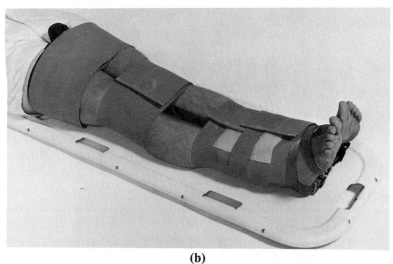

(b)

1. Position the victim on a long backboard or stretcher.
2. The first EMT supports the leg and maintains gentle traction while the second EMT cuts away the clothing and removes the shoe and sock to check the pulse and sensation at the foot.
3. Using the uninjured leg as a guide, pull the splint out to the correct length.
4. Position the splint to the inside of the injured leg with the padded bar fitted snugly against the pelvis in the groin. The splint can be used on the outside of the leg, using the strap to maintain traction against the pubis. Be very careful not to catch the genitals under the bar (or strap).
5. While maintaining gentle manual traction, attach the padded hitch to the foot and ankle.
6. Extend the splint until the correct tension is obtained.
7. Release manual traction and recheck circulation and sensation.
8. Apply elastic straps above and below the knee.

E. *Donway splint:* This is a fairly new variation of the Thomas half-ring splint. The ischial ring removes for easier attachment and traction is applied by a pneumatic pump. This splint can be applied by a single person if necessary.

1. Position the victim on a long backboard or stretcher.
2. The first EMT supports the leg and maintains gentle traction while the second EMT cuts away the clothing and removes the shoe and sock to check the pulse and sensation at the foot.
3. Feed the ischial ring under the knee, adjust around the thigh and fasten the buckle to achieve a loose fit.
4. Depress the air release valve to ensure that no excess pressure is retained in the system.
5. Unlock the collets, raise the footplate into the upright position, and place the splint over the leg.
6. Adjust the side arms of the splint to the desired length, attach to the ischial ring pegs, and lock by turning the side arms.
7. Open the ankle strap and employing the necessary support, place the patient's heel in the padded portion of the strap with the foot against the footplate.
8. Maintaining the heel against the footplate, adjust the lower Velcro attachment to ensure that the padded support member is positioned high on the ankle.
9. Crisscross the top straps tightly over the instep, starting with the longest strap.
10. Tighten the straps around the footplate and secure with the Velcro attachments.

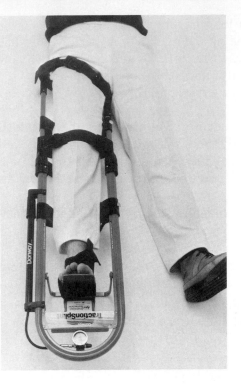

Figure S4–3. Donway Traction Splint.

11. Apply pneumatic pressure with the pump, up to the desired level of traction, and upon completion, moderately tighten the strap to secure the ring in the ischial load-bearing position. The operating range of the splint is 10 to 40 lb of traction. Safety pressure relief valves operate automatically if this range is exceeded. In this event the collets should be locked, the air released, and the normal procedure for application of traction is repeated.
12. Release manual traction and recheck circulation and sensation.
13. Align the opened leg supports with the calf and thigh. Feed the leading tapered edge under the leg, over the top of the opposite side arm and back under the leg. Adjust the tension to provide the required support and secure with the button fastener.
14. Feed the knee strap under the leg and secure above the knee with the buckle fastener.
15. As the injured leg is under traction and adequately supported, the heel stand can be raised. Recheck the traction level and adjust where necessary.
16. Turn the collets until hand tight and apply a further quarter-turn to lock the position of the side arms, and release the pneumatic pressure by depressing the air release valve until the gauge reads zero.

Skill Station 5

APPLICATION OF THE ANTISHOCK GARMENT*

Objectives

The objectives of this skill station are as follows:

1. To learn and practice the proper method of applying and inflating the antishock garment.
2. To learn and practice the proper method of deflating and removing the antishock garment.
3. To learn the indications and contraindications for the use of the antishock garment.

Caution: If these trousers are applied to live models, do not inflate them; they may cause elevations in the blood pressure.

Procedures

I. Application

A. Evaluate the victim through at least the primary survey. Apply a blood pressure cuff to his arm.

*Also known as military antishock trousers, MAST, or PASG.

B. Have the second EMT unfold the trousers and lay them flat on a long backboard and place the backboard beside the victim.

C. If shock is present, cut clothing from the lower body and perform the MAST survey.

1. Quickly examine the abdomen.
2. Feel the pelvis for stability.
3. Check the legs for injury.

D. Maintaining immobility of the spine, log-roll the victim (check the back quickly as you do this) onto the backboard. The top of the antishock garment should be just below the lowest rib.

E. Wrap the trousers around the left leg and fasten the Velcro strips.

F. Wrap the trousers around the right leg and fasten the Velcro strips.

G. Wrap the abdominal compartment around the abdomen and fasten the Velcro strips. Be sure the top of the garment is below the bottom ribs.

Figure S5–1. Application of the MAST.

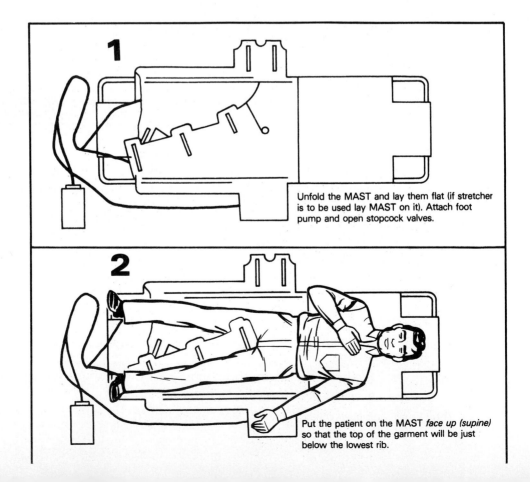

1

Unfold the MAST and lay them flat (if stretcher is to be used lay MAST on it). Attach foot pump and open stopcock valves.

2

Put the patient on the MAST *face up (supine)* so that the top of the garment will be just below the lowest rib.

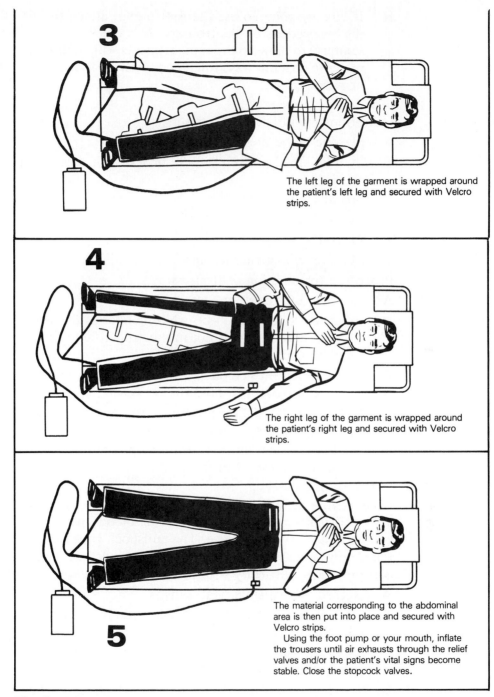

3

The left leg of the garment is wrapped around the patient's left leg and secured with Velcro strips.

4

The right leg of the garment is wrapped around the patient's right leg and secured with Velcro strips.

5

The material corresponding to the abdominal area is then put into place and secured with Velcro strips.

Using the foot pump or your mouth, inflate the trousers until air exhausts through the relief valves and/or the patient's vital signs become stable. Close the stopcock valves.

Fig. S5–1 (cont.)

203

H. If you are going to use the foot pump, attach the air tubes to the connections on the trousers. It is quicker (although not as sanitary) to blow up the compartments with your mouth; if you prefer to do it this way, you do not need the foot pump, air tubes, or gauges at all.

II. Inflation of trousers

Indications for inflation of trousers:

A. Systolic blood pressure less than 80 mmHg

B. Systolic blood pressure of 100 or less with other symptoms of shock

C. Spinal shock

D. Pelvic fractures

E. Fractures of legs

F. Massive abdominal bleeding

Procedure for inflation of trousers:

A. Recheck and record the vital signs.

B. Inflate the leg compartments while monitoring the blood pressure. If the blood pressure is not in the range 100 to 110 mmHg, inflate the abdominal compartment.

C. When the patient's blood pressure is adequate (100 to 110 mgHg), turn the stopcocks to hold the pressure.

D. Remember: It is not the pressure in the trousers you are monitoring but the pressure in the patient.

E. Continue monitoring the patient's blood pressure, adding pressure to the trousers as needed.

III. Deflation of trousers

Note: Before deflation occurs, two large-bore IVs must be inserted and sufficient volume of fluids and/or blood given to replace the volume lost from hemorrhage. The antishock garment is usually deflated only at the hospital. The only reason to deflate them in the field is if they cause difficulty with breathing (pulmonary edema).

A. Record the patient's vital signs.

B. Obtain permission to deflate the trousers from a physician knowledgeable in their use.

C. Slowly deflate the abdominal compartment while monitoring the patient's blood pressure.

D. If the blood pressure drops 5 mmHg or more, you must stop deflation and infuse more fluid or blood until the vital signs stabilize again (this usually requires at least 200 cc).

E. Proceed from the abdominal compartment to the right leg and then left leg with your deflation, continuously monitoring the blood pressure and stopping to infuse fluid when a drop of 5 mmHg occurs.

F. If the patient experiences a sudden precipitous drop in blood pressure while you are deflating, stop and reinflate the garment.

IV. **Application of antishock trousers to a victim requiring a traction splint**

A. Have your partner hold traction on the fractured leg.

B. Unfold the trousers and lay them flat on a long spine board.

C. Log-roll the victim, holding traction on the injured leg and keeping the neck stabilized.

D. Slide the spine board and the victim so that the top of the trousers is just below the lowest rib. If the victim is already on a spine board, you may simply unfold the trousers and slide them under the victim while maintaining traction on the injured leg.

E. Wrap the trousers around the injured leg and fasten the Velcro strips.

F. Wrap the trousers around the other leg and fasten the Velcro strips.

G. Wrap the abdominal compartment around the abdomen and fasten the Velcro strips. Be sure that the top of the garment is below the bottom ribs.

H. Apply a traction splint (Thomas, Hare, Sager, or Klippel) over the trousers. Attach the straps and apply traction.

I. Inflate the trousers in the usual sequence.

Important Points to Remember

1. Remove the trousers only in the hospital setting unless pulmonary edema is precipitated by application.

2. Inflate the trousers until a systolic blood pressure of 100 to 110 mmHg is obtained.

3. Monitor vital signs frequently.

4. During deflation, a blood pressure drop of 5 mmHg signals that deflation must stop until more fluids are replaced.

5. Never allow deflation of the antishock garment by personnel inexperienced in its use.

6. Never deflate the antishock trousers without adequate volume replacement and a good intravenous route established.

7. Never deflate the entire garment at once.
8. Never deflate the legs before the abdomen.
9. Do not allow anyone to cut the garment.
10. If necessary, patients may go to surgery with the garment in place.

Review

I. **Indications for use of antishock trousers**
    A. Systolic blood pressure less than 80 mmHg
    B. Systolic blood pressure of 100 or less with other symptoms of shock
    C. Spinal shock
    D. Pelvic fractures
    E. Fractures of legs
    F. Spinal shock
    G. Massive abdominal bleeding

II. **Contraindications for use of antishock trousers**
    A. Absolute: pulmonary edema
    B. Conditional
        1. *Pregnancy:* May use leg compartments.
        2. *Abdominal injury with protruding viscera:* Use leg compartments.
        3. *Penetrating chest wounds with shock:* Do not attempt to raise the blood pressure above 100 mmHg systolic; you may increase intrathoracic bleeding.

Skill Station 6

HELMET REMOVAL

Objectives

The objective of this skill station is to learn and practice how to remove a helmet without injuring the spine.

Procedures

I. **Removing a helmet from a victim with a possible cervical spine injury**
   A. The first EMT positions himself above or behind the victim, places his hands on each side of the helmet, and immobilizes the head and neck by holding the helmet and the victim's neck.
   B. The second EMT positions himself to the side of the victim and removes the chin strap. Chin straps can usually be removed easily without cutting them.
   C. The second EMT then assumes the stabilization by placing one hand under the neck at the occiput and the other hand on the anterior neck with the thumb pressing on one angle of the mandible and the index and middle fingers pressing on the other angle of the mandible.

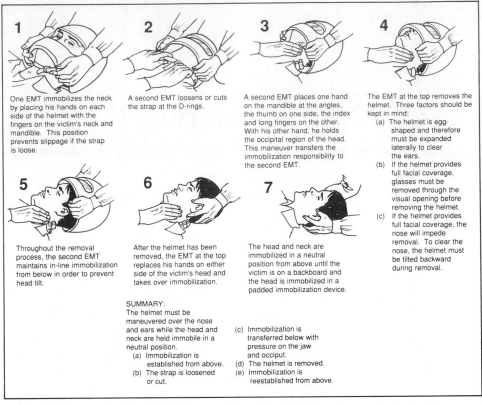

Figure S6–1. Helmet removal from injured patient.

D.   The first EMT now removes the helmet by pulling out laterally on each side to clear the ears and then up to remove. Full-face helmets will have to be tilted back to clear the nose (tilt the helmet, not the head). If the victim is wearing glasses, the first EMT should remove them through the visual opening before removing the full-face helmet. The second EMT maintains steady immobilization of the neck during this procedure.

E.   After removal of the helmet, the first EMT takes over the neck immobilization again by grasping the head on either side with his fingers holding the angle of the jaw and the occiput.

F.   The second EMT now applies a suitable cervical immobilization device.

II.   Alternate procedure for removing a helmet
This has the advantage of one EMT maintaining immobilization of the neck throughout the whole procedure. This procedure does not work well with full-face helmets.

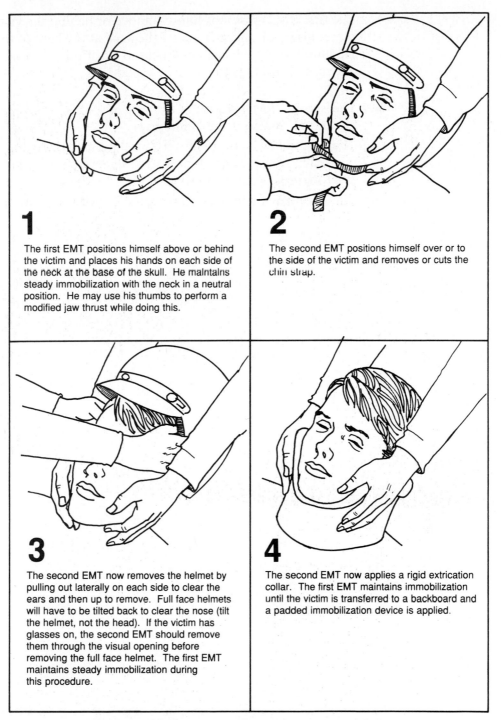

1

The first EMT positions himself above or behind the victim and places his hands on each side of the neck at the base of the skull. He maintains steady immobilization with the neck in a neutral position. He may use his thumbs to perform a modified jaw thrust while doing this.

2

The second EMT positions himself over or to the side of the victim and removes or cuts the chin strap.

3

The second EMT now removes the helmet by pulling out laterally on each side to clear the ears and then up to remove. Full face helmets will have to be tilted back to clear the nose (tilt the helmet, not the head). If the victim has glasses on, the second EMT should remove them through the visual opening before removing the full face helmet. The first EMT maintains steady immobilization during this procedure.

4

The second EMT now applies a rigid extrication collar. The first EMT maintains immobilization until the victim is transferred to a backboard and a padded immobilization device is applied.

Figure S6–2. Alternate method for removal of helmet.

A. The first EMT positions himself above or behind the victim and places his hands on each side of the neck at the base of the skull. He immobilizes the neck in a neutral position. If necessary, he may use his thumbs to perform a modified jaw thrust while doing this.

B. The second EMT positions himself over or to the side of the victim and removes the chin strap.

C. The second EMT now removes the helmet by pulling out laterally on each side to clear the ears and then up to remove. The first EMT maintains immobilization of the neck during the procedure.

D. The second EMT now applies a suitable cervical immobilization device.

Skill Station 7

LONG BACKBOARD

Objectives

The objectives of this skill station are as follows:

1. To learn and practice logrolling a victim onto a long backboard.
2. To learn and practice securing a victim to a long backboard.
3. To learn and practice immobilizing a victim from a standing position.
4. To learn and practice immobilizing the head and neck when a neutral position cannot safely be attained.

Procedures

I. **Logrolling the supine victim**
   A. EMT number 1 maintains the spine immobilized in a neutral position. A rigid extrication collar is applied. Even with the collar in place, EMT 1 maintains the head and neck in a neutral position until the log-rolling maneuver is completed.
   B. The victim is placed with his legs extended in the normal manner and his arms (palms inward) extended by his sides. The victim will be rolled up on one arm with that arm acting as a splint for the body.

211

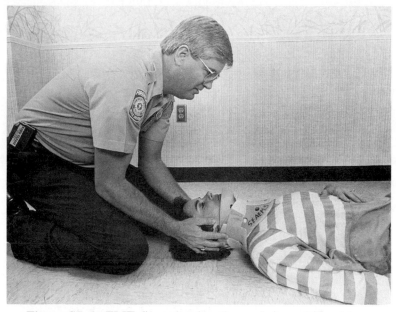

Figure S7–1. EMT #1 maintains the neck immobilized in a neutral position.

C. The long backboard is positioned next to the body. If one arm is injured, place the backboard on the injured side so that the victim will roll upon the uninjured arm.

D. EMTs 2 and 3 kneel at the victim's side opposite the board.

E. EMT 2 is positioned at the midchest area and EMT 3 is by the upper legs.

F. EMT 2 with his knees, holds the victim's near arm in place. He then reaches across the victim and grasps the shoulder and the hips, holding the victim's far arm in place. Usually, it is possible to grasp the victim's clothing to help with the roll.

G. EMT 3, with one hand reaches across the victim and grasps the hip. With his other hand, he holds the feet together at the lower legs.

H. EMT 2, when everyone is ready, gives the order to roll the victim.

I. EMT 1 carefully keeps the head and neck in a neutral position (anterior-posterior as well as laterally) during the roll.

J. EMTs 2 and 3 roll the victim up on his side toward them. The victim's arms are kept locked to his side to maintain a splinting effect. The head, shoulders, and pelvis are kept in line during the roll.

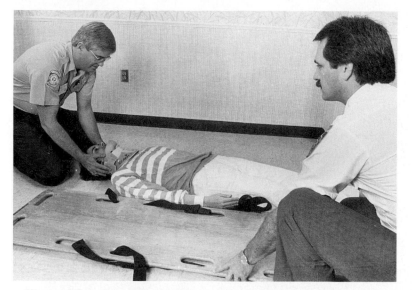

Figure S7-2. The long backboard is positioned beside the victim. Note that the straps are already laced into the correct holes in preparation for securing the victim.

Figure S7-3. EMT #2 and EMT #3 assume their positions at the victim's side opposite the board.

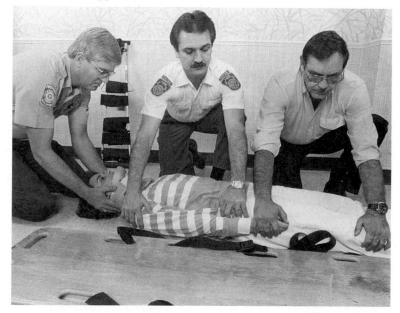

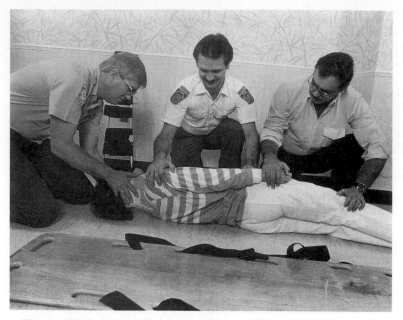

Figure S7-4. The victim is carefully rolled upon his/her side.

K. When the victim is upon his/her side, EMT 2 (or EMT4, if available) quickly examines the back for injuries.

L. The backboard is now positioned next to the victim and held at a 30 to 45 degree angle by EMT 4. If there are only three EMTs, the board is pulled into place by EMT 2 or 3. The board is left flat in this case.

M. When everybody is ready, EMT 2 gives the order to roll the victim onto the backboard. This is accomplished keeping head, shoulders, and pelvis in line.

II. **Logrolling the prone (face down) victim**

The status of the airway is critical for decisions concerning the order of the log-rolling procedure. There are three clinical situations that dictate how you should proceed.

1. The victim who is not breathing or who is in severe respiratory difficulty must be log-rolled immediately in order to manage the airway. Unless the backboard is already positioned, you must log-roll the victim, manage the airway, then transfer the victim to the backboard (in a second logrolling step) when ready to transport.

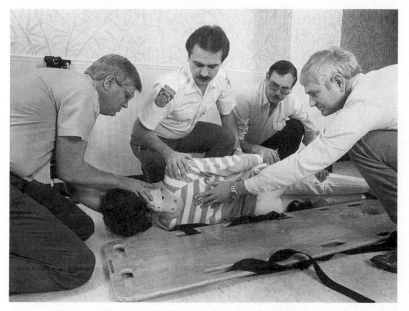

Figure S7–5. Quickly examine the back for injuries.

Figure S7–6A. If another EMT is available, he positions the backboard next to the victim at a 30-45 degree angle.

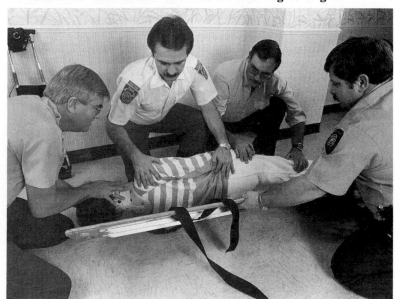

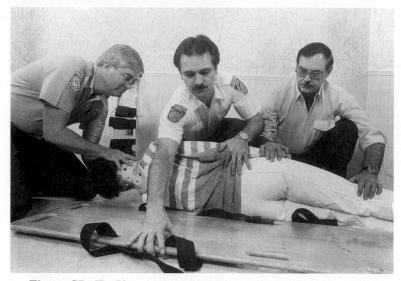

Figure S7–6B. If no other help is available EMT #2 or #3 positions the backboard and leaves it flat.

Figure S7–7. At EMT #2's order, the victim is rolled onto the backboard. All movements are coordinated so that the spine is kept straight at all times.

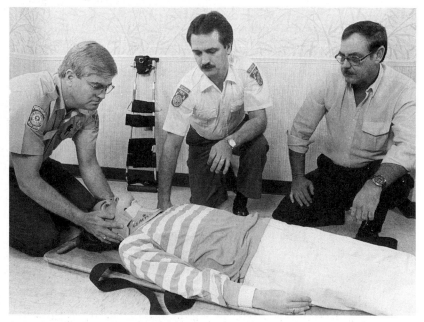

2. The victim with profuse bleeding of the mouth or nose must not be turned to the supine position. Profuse upper airway bleeding in a supine victim is a guarantee of aspiration. This victim will have to be carefully immobilized and transported prone or on his side, allowing gravity to help keep the airway clear.

3. The victim with an adequate airway and respiration should be log-rolled directly onto a backboard.

The procedure to log-roll the supine victim who has an adequate airway is as follows:

A. EMT 1 immobilizes the neck in a neutral position. When placing the hands on the head and neck, the EMT's thumbs always point toward the victim's face. This prevents having the EMT's arms crossed when the victim is log-rolled. A rigid extrication collar is applied.

B. A rapid survey is done (including the back) and the victim is placed with his legs extended in the normal manner and his arms (palms inward) extended by his sides. The victim will be rolled up on one arm, with that arm acting as a splint for the body.

C. The long backboard is positioned next to the body. The backboard is placed on the side of EMT 1's lower hand (if EMT 1's lower hand is on the victim's right side, the backboard is placed on the victim's right side). If the arm next to the backboard is injured, carefully raise the arm above the victim's head so he does not roll on the injured arm.

D. EMTs 2 and 3 kneel at the victim's side opposite the board.

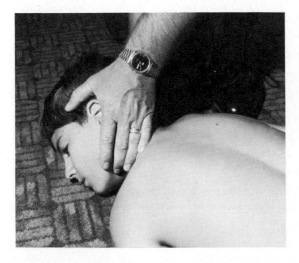

Figure S7–8. When immobilizing the neck of the prone (or supine) victim, your thumbs always point toward the face (not the occiput). This prevents having your arms crossed when the victim is rolled over.

E. EMT 2 is positioned at the midchest area and EMT 3 is by the upper legs.

F. EMT 2 grasps the shoulder and the hip. Usually, it is possible to grasp the victim's clothing to help with the roll.

G. EMT 3 grasps the hip (holding the near arm in place) and the lower legs (holding them together).

H. EMT 2, when everyone is ready, gives the order to roll the victim.

I. EMT 1 carefully keeps the head and neck in a neutral position (anteroposterior as well as laterally) during the roll.

J. EMTs 2 and 3 roll the victim up on his side away from them. The victim's arms are kept locked to his side to maintain a splinting effect. The head, shoulders, and pelvis are kept in line during the roll.

K. The backboard is now positioned next to the victim and held at a 30- to 45-degree angle by EMT 4. If there are only three EMTs, the board is pulled into place by EMT 2 or 3. The board is left flat in this case.

L. When everyone is ready, EMT 2 gives the order to roll the victim onto the backboard. This is accomplished keeping the head, shoulders, and pelvis in line.

III. Securing the victim to the backboard

There are several different methods of securing the victim using straps. Two of the best commercial devices for full body immobilization are the Reeves sleeve and the Miller body splint. The Reeves sleeve is a heavy-duty sleeve that a standard backboard will slide into. Attached to this sleeve are:

1. A head immobilization device

2. Heavy vinyl-coated nylon panels that go over the chest and abdomen and are secured with seat-belt-type straps and quick-release connectors

3. Two full-length leg panels to secure the lower extremities

4. Straps to hold the arms in place beside the victim

5. Six handles for carrying the victim

6. Metal rings (2500-lb strength) for lifting the victim by rope

When the victim is in this device, he remains immobilized when lifted horizontally, vertically, or even carried on his side (like a suitcase). This device is excellent for the confused, combative victim who must be restrained for his safety.

The Miller body splint is a combination backboard, head immobilizer, and body immobilizer. Like the Reeves sleeve, it does an excellent

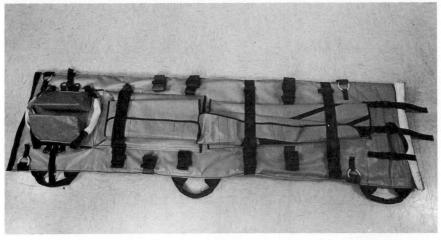

(a)

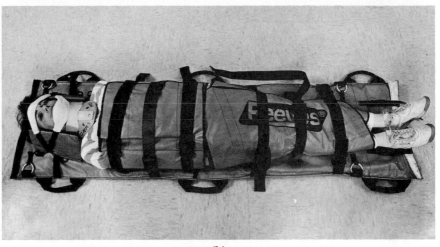

(b)

Figure S7–9A. The Reeves Sleeve.

Figure S7–9B. A victim immobilized on a Reeves Sleeve. The arms can be positioned inside the vinyl panels, between the panels and the straps, or outside the panels and the straps.

job of full-body immobilization with a minimum of time and effort.

The procedure for securing the victim to the long backboard using straps. (straps 12 ft in length are preferred) is as follows:

A. The head and neck are held in a neutral position (a rigid collar should already be in place) while padding is placed behind the head to maintain this position. A blanket roll or commercial head immobilizer are applied and strapped into position using elastic

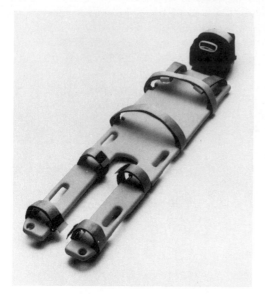

Figure S7–10. The Miller Body Splint.®

wraps or wide tape. Do not use chin straps unless they can be applied to the chin portion of the extrication collar itself. Chin straps that hold the victim's mouth closed guarantee aspiration if the victim vomits.

B. Two straps are laced through the top two lateral holes of the backboard. Apply them so that they connect together across the chest below the armpits.

C. Bring the other ends of the straps over the shoulders and across the chest.

D. Lace the straps through the lateral holes at the level of the pelvis.

E. Bring the straps back across the lower pelvis and upper legs, then lace through the lateral holes and connect below the knees. The straps must be applied quite snug so that the body does not move if the board has to be turned to allow the victim to vomit.

Nine-foot straps will work but are usually too short to go below the knees. If you use two 9-ft straps, most adults will require another strap below the knees.

IV. **Applying and securing a long backboard to a standing victim**
Method I

A. One EMT stands behind the victim and immobilizes the head and neck in a neutral position. A rigid extrication collar is applied. The EMT continues to maintain stabilization in a neutral position.

B. A long backboard is placed on the ground behind the victim.

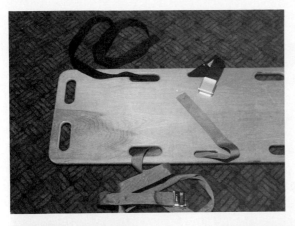

Figure S7-11 (A & B). Victim on backboard with lower end of straps connected below the armpits. The upper ends of the straps are pulled over the shoulders. Note that the victim should have his neck immobilized either manually or by an immobilization device.

(a)

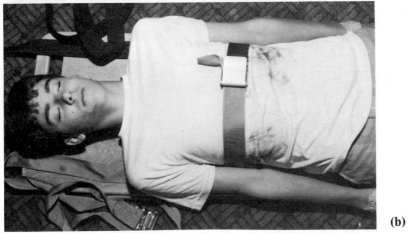

(b)

Figure S7-12. Bring the straps over the shoulders and across the chest. Lace the straps through the lateral holes at the level of the pelvis.

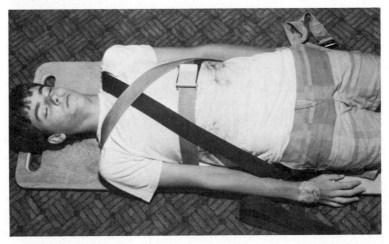

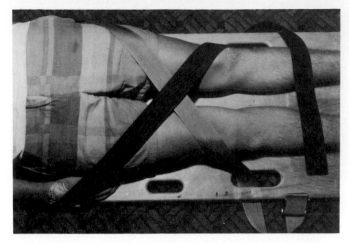

(a)

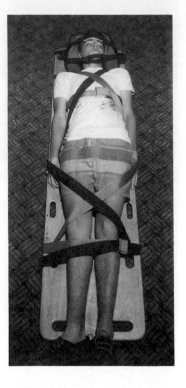

(b)

Figure S7-13A. Bring the straps back across the lower pelvis and upper legs, then lace through the lateral holes and connect below the knees.
Figure S7-13B. The straps should be tight enough to prevent any movement in case the board has to be tilted. Note that the chin strap should not be applied as shown here.

C. Other EMTs stabilize the shoulders and trunk and allow the victim to carefully sit down on the backboard.

D. The victim is carefully lowered back onto the backboard maintaining stabilization of the head, neck, and trunk.

E. The victim is centered on the backboard and secured.

Method II

A. EMT 1 stands in front of the victim and immobilizes the head and neck in a neutral position. A suitable cervical collar is applied. EMT 1 continues to maintain stabilization in a neutral position.

B. EMT 2 places a long backboard against the victim's back.

C. EMT 3 secures the victim to the board using nylon straps. These must cross over the shoulders and the pelvis and legs to prevent movement when the board is tilted down.

D. Padding is placed behind the head to maintain a neutral position and a blanket roll or commercial head immobilizer is applied and secured using elastic wraps or wide tape.

    E. The board is carefully tilted back onto a stretcher and the legs secured and feet tied together.

V. **Immobilizing the head and neck when a neutral positon cannot safely be attained**

If the head or neck is held in an angulated position and the victim complains of pain on any attempt to straighten it, you should immobilize it in the position found. The same is true of the unconscious victim whose neck is held to one side and does not easily straighten with gentle traction. You cannot use a cervical collar or commercial head immobilizer in this situation. You must use pads or a blanket roll and careful taping to immobilize the head and neck in the position found.

Skill Station 8

PRIMARY SURVEY

Objectives

The objectives of this skill station are as follows:

1. To learn to perform the primary survey correctly.
2. To learn which patients require "load and go."
3. To learn when to perform critical interventions.

Conducting the Primary Survey

This is a rapid exam to determine life-threatening conditions. The information that you gather here is used to make decisions about critical interventions and time of transport. This exam should not take over $1\frac{1}{2}$ to 2 minutes. This exam is so important that nothing is allowed to interrupt it except airway obstruction or cardiac arrest. Respiratory distress (other than airway obstruction) is not an indication to interrupt the primary survey because the cause of respiratory distress is frequently found during examination of the chest. Major bleeding is also controlled at this time.

Assessment Priorities

A. *Primary survey*
1. Evaluate *Airway,* C-spine control, and initial level of consciousness.
2. Evaluate *Breathing.*
3. Evaluate *Circulation.*
4. Stop major *bleeding.*

B. *Transport decision and critical interventions*

C. *Secondary survey*
1. Vital signs
2. History of patient and trauma event
3. Head-to-toes exam (including neurological)
4. Further bandaging and splinting
5. Continual monitoring

These steps must be memorized until you can perform them in the correct sequence without stopping to think about what comes next. They are the ABCs of Basic Trauma Life Support.

Patient Assessment Using the Priority Plan

Once you approach the victim, your exam should proceed quickly and smoothly. Unless held up by extrication, on-scene time should be under 10 minutes. Critical victims should have on-scene times of 5 minutes or less. Nothing interrupts the primary survey except treatment of airway obstruction or cardiac arrest.

A. *Evaluate airway, C-spine control, and initial LOC (level of consciousness).* Assessment begins immediately, even if the victim is being extricated. Extrication should not interfere with patient care. The same priorities apply continually before, during, and after extrication. The team leader should approach the victim from the front (face to face, so that he does not turn his head to see you). A second EMT immediately, gently, but firmly, stabilizes the neck in a neutral position. He must not release his hold on the neck until someone relieves him or a suitable stabilization device is applied. The team leader should say to the patient: "We are EMTs here to help you. What happened? The patient's reply gives immediate information about both the airway and the level of consciousness. If the patient responds appropriately to your ques-

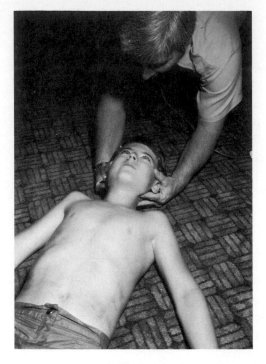

**Figure S8–1. Your partner
should immediately immobilize
the neck in a neutral position.**

tion, you have established that he has an open airway and his level
of consciousness is normal. If the patient cannot speak or is unconscious, you must further evaluate the airway. Look, listen, and
feel for movement of air. Open the mouth and clear the airway if
necessary. If the airway is obstructed, use the appropriate method to
open before finishing the primary survey. Because of the ever-present
danger of spinal injury, you must never extend the neck to open the
airway of a trauma patient. Patients with airway difficulty or decreased
level of consciousness are in the rapid transport category. All patients
with decreased LOC should get oxygen and hyperventilation (24 breaths
per minute). Your partner may use his knees to maintain immobilization of the neck, freeing his hands to apply oxygen or use a
bag–valve–mask to assist ventilation. This is another reason that all
equipment should be within immediate reach. If you assist ventilation, be sure that the patient not only gets an adequate ventilatory
rate, but also an adequate volume with each breath.

B. *Assess breathing and circulation:* It is impractical to separate evaluation of breathing and circulation since you must check both as you
quickly look, listen, and feel the neck and chest. There is much infor-

mation to be gained when this examination is performed correctly. (*Remember:* If the patient is not breathing, you must immediately give two full breaths and then check for a carotid pulse. If there is no pulse, you must begin cardiopulmonary resuscitation.) After your partner has immobilized the neck and (if necessary) opened the airway with a modified jaw thrust, you should proceed with evaluation of breathing and circulation in the following manner.

1. Place your face over the patient's mouth so that you can judge both the rate and quality of breathing. Is breathing too fast (>24 per minute) or too slow (<12 per minute)? Is the victim moving an adequate volume of air when he breathes? Any abnormality of breathing signals a search for the cause as well as administration of oxygen and possibly breathing assistance. Your partner can apply the nonbreather oxygen mask or bag–valve device without interrupting your survey.

2. As your partner holds the neck stable, he will find that it is simple to feel the carotid pulse with his index finger. He should note rate and quality, then compare with your evaluation of the pulse at the wrist. Also evaluate skin color/condition and capillary refill. This information, combined with LOC, is the best early assessment of circulatory status and the presence of shock. If the pulse is present at the neck and the wrist, the blood pressure is greater than 80 mmHg (it may be normal—judge by the strength of the pulse—it is not yet time to use the blood pressure cuff). If the pulse is present at the neck but not at the wrist, the blood pressure is between 60 and 80 mmHg. This means *late* shock. Even if the pulse is present and strong at the neck and wrist, you may be able to diagnose *early* shock by other signs. Other signs of shock include slow capillary refill, rapid heart rate (>100 per minute), cold sweaty skin, pale appearance, confusion, weakness, or thirst. *Remember:* The patient with spinal shock may not be pale, cold, or sweaty and will not have a rapid pulse. He will have a low blood pressure and paralysis. All patients with shock should get oxygen and should have the antishock garment applied as soon as they are on the backboard.

3. As soon as you have noted the breathing and pulse, quickly look and feel to determine if the trachea is in the midline, if the neck veins are flat or distended, and if there is discoloration or swelling. You may apply a rigid extrication collar at this time.

4. Now look, feel, and listen to the chest. If there is any difficulty with respiration, the chest must be bared for examination: This

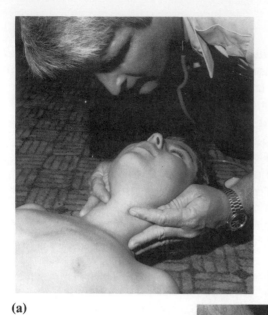

Figure S8–2A. Your partner feels the carotid pulse.

Figure S8–2B. Compare the carotid pulse with your evaluation of the pulse at the wrist.

Figure S8–2C. Check capillary refill.

(a)

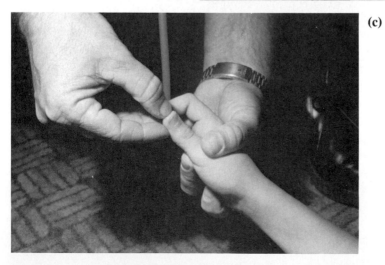

(b)

(c)

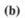

is no time for modesty; chest injuries often kill quickly. Look for sucking chest wounds, flail segments, contusions, or deformities. Note if the ribs rise with respiration or if there is only diaphragmatic breathing. Feel for instability, tenderness, or crepitation. Listen for breath sounds. Are they *present and equal* on both sides? If breath sounds are not equal (decreased or absent on one side), you should determine if tension pneumothorax is present. If abnormalities are found here (open chest wound, flail chest, respiratory difficulty), you should make the appropriate

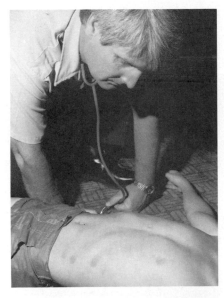

Figure S8–3A. Look for penetrating wounds, flail segments, contusions, or deformities.
Figure S8–3B. Feel for crepitation, tenderness, or instability.
Figure S8–3C. Listen to see if breath sounds are present and equal.

(a)

(b)

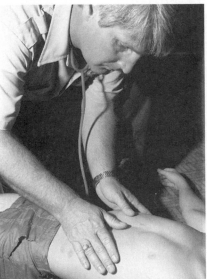

(c)

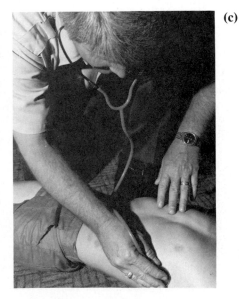

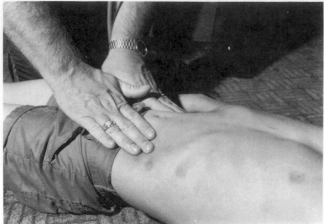

Figure S8–4A. Are there contusions, penetrations, distention, or tenderness of the abdomen?
Figure S8–4B. Is the pelvis tender or unstable?
Figure S8–4C. Is there any sign of trauma to the legs?

(a)

(b)

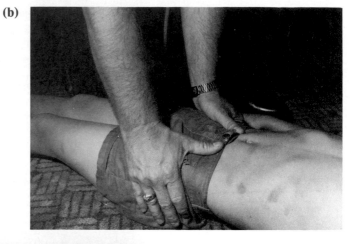

(c)

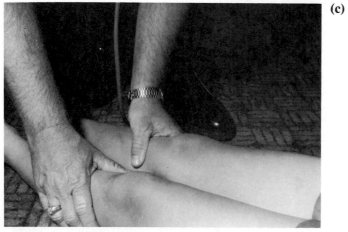

intervention (seal open wound, *hand stabilize* flail, give oxygen, assist ventilation).

5. Stop active bleeding. Your other partner should have already done this, or at least begun to do this. Almost all bleeding can be stopped by direct pressure; use gauze pads and bandage or elastic wraps. You may use air splints or antishock garment to tamponade bleeding. Tourniquets may be needed in *rare* situations. If a dressing becomes blood soaked, you may remove the dressing and redress once to be sure that you are applying pressure to the bleeding site. It is important that you report such excessive bleeding to the receiving physician. Do not use clamps to stop bleeders; you may cause injuries to other structures (nerves are present alongside arteries).

6. MAST survey. If your primary survey identified the presence of a critical situation, you should modify the primary survey by adding the MAST survey. Since a critical condition requires transport before performing the secondary survey, and you may have to apply the antishock garment (MAST, PASG) before you do the secondary survey, you need to check quickly the areas of the body that will be hidden by the garment. You must expose the body to do this. Quickly cut off clothes, maintaining body warmth and modesty with a sheet or blanket. The MAST survey consists of quickly examining the abdomen, pelvis, and legs.

At this point you have enough information to determine critical trauma situations that should be treated by "load and go."

Critical Injuries/Conditions

A. *Airway obstruction unrelieved by mechanical methods* (i.e., suction, forceps)
B. *Conditions resulting in possible inadequate breathing*
    1. Large open chest wound (sucking chest wound)
    2. Large flail chest
    3. Tension pneumothorax
    4. Major blunt chest injury
C. *Traumatic cardiopulmonary arrest*
D. *Shock*
    1. Hemorrhagic
    2. Spinal

   3. Myocardial contusion
   4. Pericardial tamponade
E. *Head injury with decreased level of consciousness*

This can be further simplified into three conditions based on signs and symptoms:

1. *Difficulty with respiration*
2. *Difficulty with circulation (shock)*
3. *Decreased level of consciousness*

Any trauma patient with one or more of these conditions falls into the "load and go" category. When you finish the primary survey, you have enough information to decide if the patient is critical or stable. If the patient has one of the critical conditions, you should immediately transfer him to a long backboard (check his back as you log-roll him), apply MAST and oxygen, load him into an ambulance (if available), and transport rapidly to the nearest appropriate emergency facility. Lifesaving procedures may be needed but should not hold up transport. There are a few brief procedures that are done while at the scene (attempt to relieve airway obstruction, seal sucking chest wound, hand stabilize flail, hyperventilate, begin CPR), but most are reserved for transport. You must weigh every field procedure against the time it will take to perform. You are spending minutes of the patient's golden hour; be sure the procedure is worth the cost. Nonlifesaving procedures (splinting and bandaging) must not hold up transport. Be sure to call medical control early so that the hospital is prepared for your arrival.

If the primary survey fails to identify a critical trauma situation, you should transfer the victim to the backboard (check the back) and proceed with the secondary survey.

Procedure

Short written scenarios will be used along with a model (to act as the victim). You will divide into teams of three to practice performing the primary survey, critical interventions, and transport decisions. The "parrot phrases" are the words you should repeat (like a parrot) at each step of the survey. These represent the answers you should be seeking at each step of the survey. Each member of the team must practice being team leader at least once and preferably twice.

THE BASIC TRAUMA LIFE SUPPORT PRIMARY SURVEY

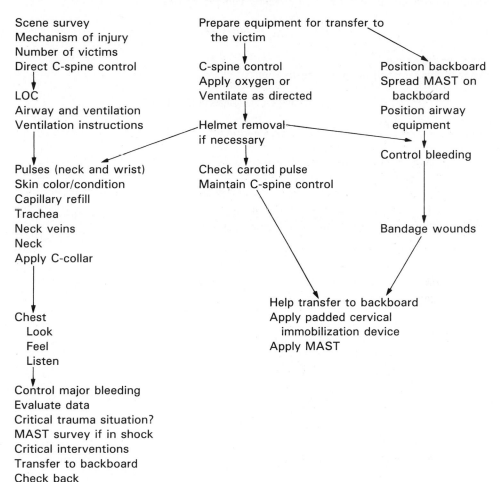

TEAM LEADER

Scene survey
Mechanism of injury
Number of victims
Direct C-spine control

LOC
Airway and ventilation
Ventilation instructions

Pulses (neck and wrist)
Skin color/condition
Capillary refill
Trachea
Neck veins
Neck
Apply C-collar

Chest
  Look
  Feel
  Listen

Control major bleeding
Evaluate data
Critical trauma situation?
MAST survey if in shock
Critical interventions
Transfer to backboard
Check back

TEAM MEMBERS

Prepare equipment for transfer to
  the victim

C-spine control
Apply oxygen or
Ventilate as directed

Helmet removal
if necessary

Check carotid pulse
Maintain C-spine control

Position backboard
Spread MAST on
  backboard
Position airway
  equipment

Control bleeding

Bandage wounds

Help transfer to backboard
Apply padded cervical
  immobilization device
Apply MAST

PARROT PHRASES

SCENE SURVEY

I am surveying the scene. Are there any dangers?
I am surveying for mechanisms of injury.
Are there any other victims?

LEVEL OF CONSCIOUSNESS

We are EMTs here to help you. What happened?
Please do not move until we have checked you for injuries.

AIRWAY

Is the airway clean?
What is the rate and quality of respiration?

VENTILATION INSTRUCTIONS

Order oxygen for any airway difficulty, head injury, or shock.
Assist ventilation if hypoventilating.
Hyperventilate altered level of consciousness.

PULSES

What is the rate and quality of the pulse at the neck and the wrist?

SKIN COLOR AND CONDITION

What is the skin color and condition?

CAPILLARY REFILL

Is the capillary refill normal or delayed?

TRACHEA

Is the trachea midline or deviated?

NECK VEINS

Are the neck veins flat or distended?

NECK

Are there signs of trauma to the neck?

CHEST

I am looking at the chest. Are there any penetrations, contusions, deformities, or paradoxical motions?

I am feeling the chest. Is there any crepitation, tenderness, or instability?

I am listening to the chest. Are the breath sounds present and equal?

If breath sounds are not equal:

I am percussing the chest. Is there hyperresonance or dullness on either side?

BLEEDING

Is there any obvious bleeding?

MAST SURVEY

ABDOMEN

Are there any contusions, penetrations, distention, or tenderness of the abdomen?

PELVIS

Is the pelvis tender or unstable?

LOWER EXTREMITIES

Is there any sign of trauma to the legs?

EXAM OF THE BACK
(done during transfer to the backboard)

Is there any sign of trauma to the back?

Skill Station 9

SECONDARY SURVEY

Objectives

The objectives of this skill station are as follows:

1. To learn to perform the secondary survey correctly.
2. To learn which patients require "load and go."
3. To learn how to communicate with medical control.

Conducting the Secondary Survey

The secondary survey is a detailed exam to pick up all injuries, both obvious and potential. This exam also establishes the baseline from which many treatment decisions will be made. Critical patients will always have this exam done during transport. If the primary survey has revealed no critical condition, perform this exam while on the scene. It is important to record this exam.

1. Check vital signs. Record pulse, respiration, and blood pressure (obtain accurate recordings and use the BP cuff now).

2. Obtain a history of the injury (your partner may already have done this).
    a. Personal observation.
    b. Bystanders.
    c. Victim. Look for a Medic Alert tag in unconscious patients. Take an AMPLE history from conscious patients:
        A   allergies
        M   medications
        P   past medical history (other illnesses)
        L   last meal (when it was eaten)
        E   events preceding the accident
3. Do a head-to-toes exam.
    a. Begin at the head examining for contusions, lacerations, raccoon eyes, Battle's sign, and drainage of blood or fluid from the ears or nose. Assess the airway again.
    b. Check the neck again. Look for lacerations, contusions, tenderness, distended neck veins, or deviated trachea. Check the pulse again. If not already done, apply a cervical immobilization device at this time.
    c. Recheck the chest. Be sure that breath sounds are still present and equal on each side. Recheck seals over open wounds. Be sure that flails are well stabilized.
    d. Examine the abdomen. Look for signs of blunt or penetrating trauma. Feel for tenderness. Do not waste time listening for bowel sounds. If the abdomen is painful to gentle pressure during examination, you can expect the patient to be bleeding internally. If the abdomen is both distended and painful, you can expect hemorrhagic shock very quickly.
    e. Assess pelvis and extremities. Be sure to check and record distal sensation and pulses on all fractures. Do this before and after straightening any fracture. Angulated fractures of the upper extremities are usually best splinted as found. Most fractures of the lower extremities are straightened by using traction splints or air splints. *Critical patients have all splints applied during transport.*

Transport immediately if your secondary survey reveals any of the following:

1. Tender, distended abdomen
2. Pelvic instability
3. Bilateral femur fractures

Even though the patient may appear stable at this time, he will probably soon develop shock because of the large blood loss that is associated with these injuries.

4. Do a brief neurological exam. The neurological exam is very simple, but is frequently forgotten. It gives important baseline information that is used in later treatment decisions. Perform and record this exam.
   a. *Level of consciousness*
      A   alert
      V   responds to verbal stimuli
      P   responds to pain
      U   unresponsive
   b. *Motor:* Can he move fingers and toes?
   c. *Sensation:* Can he feel you when you touch his fingers and toes? Does the unconscious patient respond when you pinch his fingers and toes?
   d. *Pupils:* Are they equal or unequal? Do they respond to light?
5. If necessary, finish bandaging and splinting.
6. Continually monitor and reevaluate the patient. Accurately record what you see and what you do. Record changes in the patient's condition during transport. Record the time the antishock garment or tourniquet is applied. Extenuating circumstances or significant details should be recorded in the comments or remarks section of the run report.

Contacting Medical Control

This is important so that the emergency department can be prepared for the arrival of the patient. It is extremely important to do this as early as possible when you have a patient with a critical condition. It takes time to get the appropriate surgeon and the operating room team called in. The critical victim has no time to wait. Following is the procedure to communicate with medical control:

1. Identify yourself; give level of training and organization.
2. Give the patient's approximate age, sex, mechanisms of injuries, nature of the injuries, vital signs, level of consciousness, procedures performed, and the patient's response.
3. Transport the patient to the facility named by medical control.

4.   Notify the facility of the estimated time of arrival (ETA), the condition of the patient, and any special needs on arrival.

The following pages contain a brief outline of the secondary survey as well as the thoughts that should go through your mind as you perform the survey.

Procedure

Short written scenarios will be used along with a model (to act as the victim). You will divide into teams of three to practice performing the secondary survey.

THE BASIC TRAUMA LIFE SUPPORT SECONDARY SURVEY

When performing the secondary survey, you must visualize and palpate from head to toes. Everyone gets a secondary survey: stable patients while at the scene, critical patients during transport. If other team members are available, the blood pressure and accurate pulse and respiratory rates may be taken by one of them.

HEAD

1.   Palpate
     Entire scalp for lacerations or contusions
     Face for tenderness or fractures
2.   Look
     For Battle's sign
     For blood or fluid in ears
     For raccoon eyes
     For blood or fluid from nose
     For pupillary size, equality, reaction to light
     For burns of face, nose hairs, mouth
     For skin changes
          Pallor
          Cyanosis
          Diaphoresis
          Bruising
3.   Reassess
     a.   Airway
          Check for carbonacious (sooty) sputum if burn victim
     b.   Breathing
          Rate (accurately and record)
          Quality
     c.   Circulation
          Rate (accurately and record)

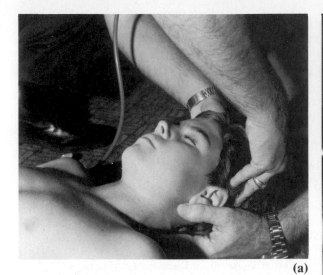

(a)

Figure S9–1A. Carefully feel scalp and face for injuries.
Figure S9–1B. Check pupils for size, equality, reaction to light.

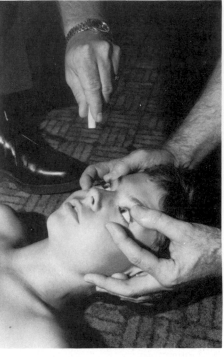

(b)

Quality
Blood pressure (done by partner if possible)

NECK (If collar has been applied, remove the front)

Signs of trauma?
JVD?
Tracheal deviation?

CHEST

Look for penetrations, contusions, deformities, or paradoxical motions
Feel for instability, tenderness, crepitation
Listen for breath sounds in all lung fields
Percuss if breath sounds unequal

ABDOMEN (If MAST has been applied, this has been completed)

Look for penetrations, contusions, distention
Palpate all four quadrants for tenderness

PELVIS (If MAST has been applied, this has been completed)

Compress laterally and over symphysis for tenderness or instability

Figure S9–2. Recheck the neck for trauma, JVD, and Tracheal deviation.

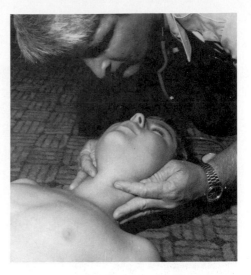

(a)

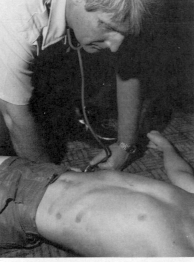

Figure S9–3A. Examine the chest for penetrations, contusions, deformities, or flail segments.
Figure S9–3B. Feel the chest for instability, tenderness, or crepitation.
Figure S9–3C. Listen to see if breath sounds are present and equal.

(b)

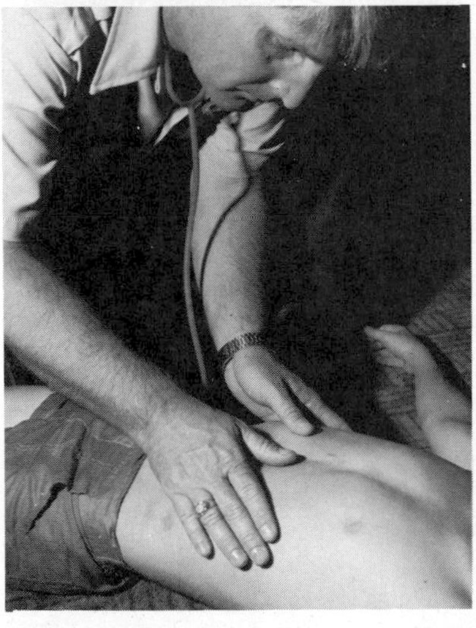

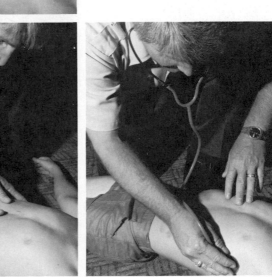

(c)

241

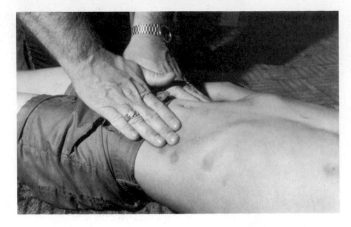

Figure S9-4. Examine the abdomen for penetrations, contusions, distention, and tenderness.

Figure S9-5. Check the pelvis for tenderness or instability.

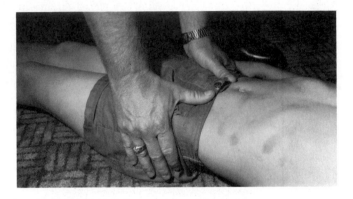

LOWER EXTREMITIES (If MAST applied, do pulses, neuro, cap refill)

Visualize and palpate for signs of trauma
Check distal pulses
Do neurological
    sensory (pinch toes)
    motor (have patient move toes)
Check range of motion
Repeat capillary refill (unless you have already made the diagnosis of shock)

UPPER EXTREMITIES

Visualize and palpate for signs of trauma
Begin at the midline, checking clavicles, shoulders, arms, and hands
Check distal pulses
Do neurological
    sensory (pinch fingers)
    motor (have patient move fingers)
Check range of motion
Repeat capillary refill (unless you have already made the diagnosis of shock)

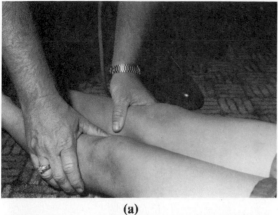

(a)

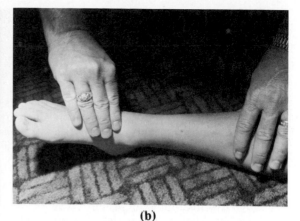

(b)

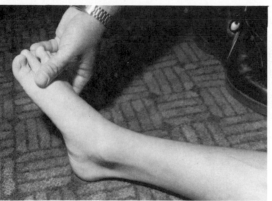

(c)

Figure S9–6A. Examine the legs for signs of trauma.
Figure S9–6B. Check range of motions and pulses.
Figure S9–6C. Check sensory, motor, and capillary refill.

Figure S9–7A. Examine arms for trauma, range of motion, pulses.
Figure S9–7B. Check arms for sensation, motor, and capillary refill.

(a)   (b)

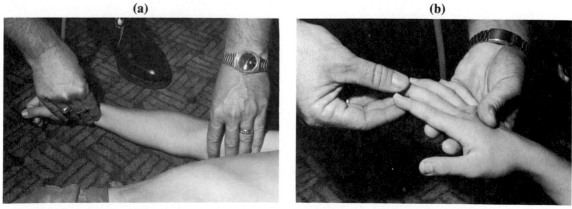

PARROT PHRASES: SECONDARY SURVEY

HEAD
I am feeling the scalp. Are there lacerations, contusions, or deformity?
I am feeling the face. Are there contusions or deformity?
Are Battle's sign or raccoon eyes present?
Is there blood or fluid draining from the ears or nose?
What is pupillary size? Are the pupils equal? Do they react to light?
Is there pallor, cyanosis, diaphoresis, or bruising?
Are there burns of the face, nose hairs, or inside the mouth?

AIRWAY
Is the airway clear?
What is the rate and quality of respiration?
Is there soot in the sputum (if a burn victim)?

CIRCULATION
What is the rate and quality of the pulse?
What is the blood pressure?
Is the capillary refill normal or delayed? (Not done if diagnosis of shock has already been made)

NECK
Are there signs of trauma to the neck?
Are the neck veins flat or distended?
Is the trachea midline or deviated?

CHEST
I am looking at the chest. Are there any penetrations, contusions, deformities, or paradoxical motion?
I am feeling the chest. Is there any crepitation, tenderness, or instability?
I am listening to the chest. Are the breath sounds present and equal?
I am percussing the chest. Is it hyperresonant or dull? (Do only if breath sounds are unequal)

ABDOMEN (If MAST has been applied, this has been completed)
I am looking at the abdomen. Are there penetrations, contusions, or distention?
I am feeling the abdomen. Is there any tenderness?

PELVIS (If MAST has been applied, this has been completed)
Is the pelvis tender or unstable?

LOWER EXTREMITIES (If MAST has been applied, do pulses, neuro, and capillary refill)
Are there any signs of trauma to the legs?
Are pulses present?
Can he feel me touch his toes?
Can he move his toes?

Is range of motion normal?
Is capillary refill normal or delayed? (Not done if diagnosis of shock has already been made)

UPPER EXTREMITIES
Is there any sign of trauma to the arms?
Are pulses present?
Can he feel me touch his fingers?
Can he move his fingers?
Is range of motion normal?
Is capillary refill normal or delayed? (not done if diagnosis of shock has already been made)

Skill Station 10

RAPID PATIENT ASSESSMENT

Objective

The objective of this skill station is to practice the proper organized sequence of evaluation and management of the multiple trauma victim.

Procedure

Short written trauma scenarios will be used along with a model (to act as the victim). Students will be divided into three member teams to practice the management of simulated trauma situations using the principles and techniques taught in the course. You will be tested in the same manner on the second day of the course. You will be expected to use all of the principles and techniques taught in this course while managing these simulated victims. Review Chapters 3 and 14 and Skill Stations 8 and 9.

Ground Rules for Teaching and Testing

1. You will be allowed to stay together in three member groups throughout the practice and testing.

2. You will have three practice scenarios. This allows each member of the team to be team leader once.
3. You will be tested as team leader once.
4. You will assist as a member of the rescue team during two scenarios in which another member is being tested as team leader. You may assist but all assessment must be done by the team leader. This gives you a total of six scenarios from which to learn: three practice, one test, two assists while others are tested.
5. Wait outside the door until the instructor comes out and gives you your scenario.
6. You will be allowed to look over your equipment before you start your exam.
7. Be sure to ask about scene hazards if not given in the scenario.
8. If you have a live model for a victim, you must talk to that person just as you would a real victim. It is best to explain what you are doing as you examine the victim. Be confident and reassuring.
9. You must ask your instructor for things you cannot find out from your model. *Example:* Blood pressure, pulse, breath sounds, etc.
10. Wounds must be dressed just as if they are real. Procedures must be done correctly (blood pressure, log-rolling, strapping, splinting, etc.)
11. If you need a piece of equipment that is not available, ask your instructor. He may allow you to simulate the equipment.
12. During practice and testing, you may go to any station but you cannot go to the same station twice.
13. You will be graded on:
    a. Assessment of the scene
    b. Assessment of the victim
    c. Management of the victim
    d. Efficient use of time
    e. Leadership
    f. Judgment
    g. Problem-solving ability
    h. Patient interaction

Patient Assessment Pearls

1. Do not approach the victim until you have done a scene survey.
2. Do not interrupt the primary survey except for:
    a. Airway obstruction or near obstruction
    b. Cardiac or respiratory arrest

3. Give ventilation instructions as soon as you assess airway and breathing.
4. Hyperventilate (about 24 breaths per minute) all victims with decreased level of consciousness.
5. Assist ventilation on anyone who is hypoventilating (8 breaths or less per minute).
6. Give oxygen to anyone with difficulty breathing, decreased LOC, or shock. If in doubt, give oxygen.
7. If the primary survey reveals that the patient has a critical situation, complete the MAST survey.
8. If absolutely necessary, certain interventions may have to be done before transport. Remember that you are trading minutes of the patient's golden hour for these procedures. Use good judgment.
9. Transfer the patient to the backboard as soon as the primary survey (and MAST survey if indicated) is completed.
10. When primary survey is completed, decide if the patient is critical or stable. Critical trauma situations:
    a. Decreased level of consciousness
    b. Difficulty with breathing
    c. Shock
11. Critical patients get a secondary survey enroute to the hospital.
12. Stable patients get a secondary survey at the scene.
13. Transport immediately if your secondary survey reveals any of the following:
    a. Tender, distended abdomen
    b. Pelvic instability
    c. Bilateral femur fractures
14. Critical patients should not have traction splints applied at the scene (it takes too long).
15. Call medical control early if you have a critical patient (other physicians may have to be called in to treat the patient).
16. Any time the patient's condition worsens, repeat the primary survey.
17. Any time you make an intervention, repeat the primary survey.
18. When you repeat the primary survey, repeat *every* step.
19. Unconscious patients cannot protect their airways.
20. Transport pregnant victims with the backboard tilted slightly to the left. Do not let them roll over onto the floor.
21. Remain calm and *think*. Your knowledge, training, and concern are the most important tools you carry.

Example of a Trauma Scenario

Situation

A young male was driving through an intersection. His automobile was hit in the driver's side by another vehicle. (This is all you would be told; you must obtain all other information by observation or by asking the instructor.)

Injuries

This is what you are expected to identify (or at least suspect, such as spinal injuries). You will not be told what the injuries are until the scenario is over.

1. Fracture of C-7, but no spinal cord injury yet
2. Flail chest on the left
3. Ruptured spleen (abdominal injury)
4. Multiple fractures of pelvis

Patient Instructions

These are instructions given to the patient in order for him to portray his injuries correctly. You will not be aware of his instructions.

Patient: You are awake and alert. If asked, you complain of pain in the left chest and "hip." Do not complain of abdominal or neck pain. If the abdomen or neck is checked, you admit to a "little" tenderness. If your neck is not immobilized or if your neck is allowed to move; become paralyzed.

Instructions to Faculty

Primary Survey

Airway open, initial respiratory rate 24 per minute and shallow
Pulse is rapid but strong, present at neck and wrist
Capillary refill delayed
Patient diaphoretic
Neck veins flat, trachea midline
Unstable rib segment on the left
Breath sounds bilateral and equal

MAST Survey

Slight LUQ tenderness of abdomen
Pelvis tender and unstable
Legs normal

Secondary Survey

Head normal
Patient still alert, pupils midposition, equal, and reactive to light
Airway open, respiratory rate 24 per minute and shallow
Pulse 120 per minute and strong, present at neck and wrist
Capillary refill delayed
Blood pressure 120/90
Neck veins flat
Trachea midline
Chest unchanged
Arms normal, pulses normal, sensation and motor normal
Abdomen slightly more tender
Pelvis should not be examined again (would cause further internal bleeding)
Legs unchanged, pulses present, sensation and motor normal, capillary refill delayed
During transport there will be a condition change
Patient becomes poorly responsive (verbal stimuli)
Pulse 150 per minute, respiration 30 per minute and shallow, BP 70/40

Grade Sheet

This is the sheet used by the instructor to grade you.
Student's name _____
Practice _____ Test _____
Time began evaluation _____
Surveys scene and notes mechanisms of injury _____
Has partner immobilize the neck _____
Talks to victim—notes normal level of consciousness _____
Checks airway _____
Checks breathing _____
Checks pulse at the wrist, has partner check at the neck _____
Checks capillary refill _____

Checks neck veins _____

Checks trachea _____

Checks chest _____

Recognizes flail _____

Stabilizes flail (may wait until victim is extricated) _____

Extricates properly onto long backboard _____

Stabilizes flail if not already done (KED will stabilize) _____

Orders oxygen by nonrebreathing mask _____

Completes MAST survey _____

Recognizes abdominal tenderness _____

         unstable pelvis _____

Checks for bleeding _____

Time primary survey completed _____

Makes decision to "load and go" _____

Knows why—respiratory problem and probable early shock _____

Applies padded cervical immobilization device _____

Applies MAST (may inflate to stabilize the pelvis) _____

Securely straps patient to the spine board _____

Transports _____

Time of transport _____

Calls medical control and describes situation correctly _____

Monitors vital signs _____

Recognizes change in condition (shock) _____

Repeats the primary survey _____

Inflates MAST if not already inflated _____

Calls medical control and advises of change in condition _____

Performed organized primary survey   Yes _____ No _____

Interacted well with victim   Yes _____ No _____

Performed organized secondary survey   Yes _____ No _____

Efficient utilization of time   Yes _____ No _____

Displayed leadership and teamwork   Yes _____ No _____

OVERALL GRADE

Excellent—instructor potential _____

Good _____

Adequate _____

Inadequate _____

Comments _____

_____

Instructor _____

RAPID PATIENT ASSESSMENT
I.   Scene survey
II.   Carry all essential equipment as you approach the victim
III. Evaluate the victim

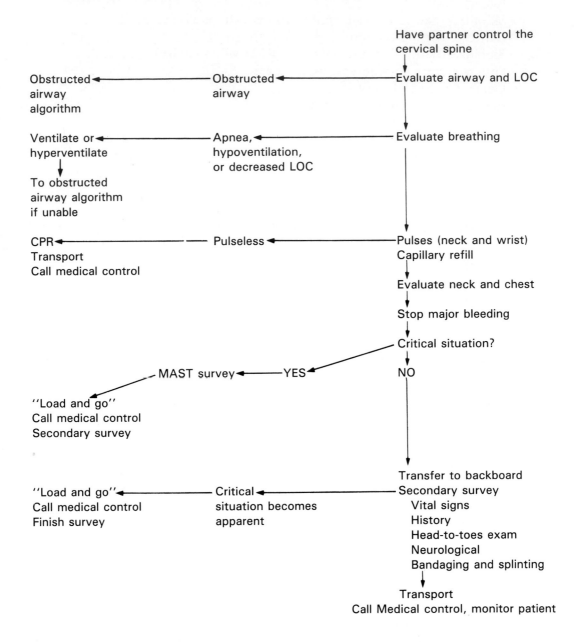

OBSTRUCTED AIRWAY ALGORITHM

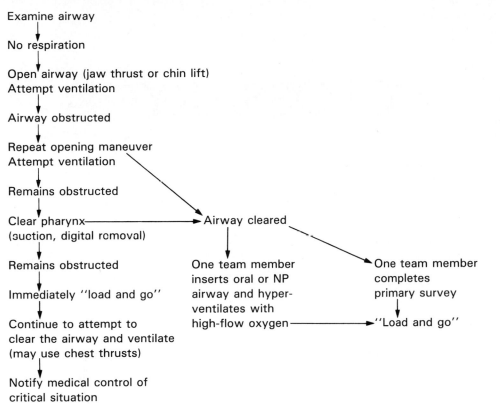

Examine airway

No respiration

Open airway (jaw thrust or chin lift)
Attempt ventilation

Airway obstructed

Repeat opening maneuver
Attempt ventilation

Remains obstructed

Clear pharynx———————————▶Airway cleared
(suction, digital removal)

Remains obstructed   One team member   One team member
                                        inserts oral or NP   completes
Immediately "load and go"   airway and hyper-   primary survey
                                        ventilates with
Continue to attempt to   high-flow oxygen————————▶"Load and go"
clear the airway and ventilate
(may use chest thrusts)

Notify medical control of
critical situation

Adapted from *An Algorithm for Rapid Assessment of the Airway* by Daniel L. Cavallaro and Patricia
J. Mominee

GLOSSARY

ABRUPTIO PLACENTA: early separation of the placenta from the uterus.

ACIDOSIS: condition caused by accumulation of acid or loss of base from the body.

AEROBIC: requiring oxygen.

ALKALOSIS: pathologic condition resulting from accumulation of base or loss of acid in the body.

ANAEROBIC: lacking oxygen.

ANOXIA: absence of oxygen supply to the tissue.

ANTISHOCK GARMENT: military antishock trousers (MAST) or pneumatic antishock garment (PASG).

ASPHYXIA: condition due to lack of oxygen, suffocation.

ASPIRATE: taking foreign matter into the lungs during inhalation.

ASSESSMENT: to evaluate the condition of a patient.

AVPU: level of consciousness (i.e., A, alert; V, responds to verbal stimuli; P, responds to pain; U, unresponsive).

AVULSION: injury in which a piece of structure is torn away.

BATTLE'S SIGN: swelling and discoloration behind the ear caused by a fracture of the base of the skull.

BRONCHOSPASM: contraction of the smooth muscle of the bronchi.

BVM (BAG–VALVE MASK): system of artificial ventilation in which the oxygen inflow fills a bag that is attached to a mask by a one-way valve.

CAPILLARY BLANCH OR REFILL: test for impairment of circulation: pressure on tip of the nail will cause the bed to turn white; if it does not turn pink again by the time it takes to say "capillary refill," the circulation is impaired.

CARBONACEOUS SPUTUM: sputum that is "sooty" or black.

CATECHOLAMINES: group of chemicals of similar structure that act to increase heart rate and blood pressure.

CENTRAL CORD SYNDROME: injury to the spinal cord that produces more loss of sensory and motor function in the arms than in the legs.

CEREBRAL PERFUSION: blood flow to the brain.

CONCUSSION: jarring injury to the brain resulting in disturbance of brain function.

CONSTRICTED: to shrink or contract.

CONTRACOUP: injury to the brain on the opposite side of the original blow.

CONTUSION: bruising; the reaction of soft tissue to a direct blow.

COUP: injury to the brain on the same side as the original blow.

CREPITATION: feeling of crackling; the sensation of fragments of broken bones rubbing together.

CUSHING REFLEX: reflex whereby the body reacts to increased pressure on the brain by raising the blood pressure.

DECELERATION: to come to a sudden stop, decreasing speed.

DERMIS: inner layer of the skin, containing hair follicles, sweat glands, sebaceous glands, nerve endings, and blood vessels.

DIAPHORESIS: to perspire profusely.

DOLL'S EYES: oculocephalic reflex; a test of brainstem function that is never performed in the prehospital setting.

DURA: tough fibrous membrane forming the outermost of the three coverings of the brain.

EGTA: esophageal gastric tube airway; an improved EOA.

EOA: esophageal obturator airway.

EPIDERMIS: outermost layer of skin.

EPIDURAL: outside the dura; between the dura and the skull.

ET TUBE: endotracheal tube.

EVISERATION: protruding of internal organs through a wound.

EXSANGUINATE: to bleed to death.

FORAMEN: an opening.

FULL THICKNESS: third-degree burn.

GENIOGLOSSUS: muscle that pulls the tongue out of the mouth.

GRUNTING: deep, gutteral noise made in breathing; a sign of respiratory distress in small children.

HARE SPLINT: type of traction splint.

HEIMLICH MANEUVER: method of dislodging food or other material from the throat of a choking victim.

HEMOTHORAX: presence of blood in the chest cavity within the pleural space, outside the lung.

HYPERRESONANT: giving an increased vibrant sound on percussion.

HYPOVOLEMIC SHOCK: hemmorrhagic shock; shock caused by insufficient blood or fluid within the body.

HYPOXIA: deficiency of oxygen reaching the tissues of the body.

INTRAABDOMINAL: within the abdomen.

INTRACRANIAL: within the skull.

INTRATHORACTIC: within the chest.

JVD: jugular vein distention.

KINEMATICS: phase of mechanics that deals with possible motions of the body.

KLIPPEL SPLINT: type of traction splint.

LOC: level of consciousness.

MAST: military antishock trousers, antishock garment, or pneumatic antishock garment (PASG).

MEDIAL: toward the middle.

MEDICAL CONTROL: physician who assumes responsibility and gives orders for individual patients in the prehospital phase of patient care.

MORTALITY: frequency of death or death rate.

NP AIRWAY: nasopharyngeal airway; an artificial airway positioned in the nasal cavity.

OCCULT INJURIES: hidden or concealed from view injuries.

PALLOR: paleness, absence of skin color.

PALPATE: to examine by touch.

PARADOXICAL MOTION: motion of the injured segment of a flail chest, opposite to the normal motion of the chest wall.

PARTIAL-THICKNESS BURN: burn that does not injure the full thickness of the skin. A first-degree burn involves only the epidermal layer. A second-degree burn involves the epidermis and part of the dermis.

PASG: pneumatic antishock garment, or military antishock trousers (MAST).

PATHOPHYSIOLOGY: basic processes of the disease.

PERFUSION: blood flow to an organ.

PIA MATER: innermost of the three layers of tissue that envelop the brain.

PLACENTA PREVIA: abnormal location of the placenta, so that it covers the opening of the uterus (cervical os).

PNEUMOTHORAX: presence of air within the chest cavity in the pleural space, but outside the lung (collapsed lung).

PULSE PRESSURE: sensation given by the heart contraction to the palpating finger.

RACCOON EYES: swelling and discoloration around both eyes; a late sign of basilar skull fracture.

RTSS: ratio telephone switch station; a type of radio that accesses the telephone lines.

SAGER SPLINT: type of traction splint.

SNORING: to breathe in a hoarse, rough noise, usually with the mouth open.

SPONTANEOUS PNEUMOTHORAX: collapsed lung caused by the rupture of a congentially weak area on the surface of the lung.

STRIDOR: breathing that has a high-pitched, harsh noise; a sign of impending airway obstruction.

STROKE VOLUME: amount of blood pumped by the heart in one beat.

SUBCUTANEOUS EMPHYSEMA: presence of air in soft tissues, giving a very characteristic crackling sensation on palpation; the "rice krispies" feeling.

TACHYPNEA: respiratory rate of 24 or more.

TAMPONADE: compression of a part of the anatomy, as the compression of heart by pericardial fluid.

TENSION PNEUMOTHORAX: condition in which air continuously leaks out of the lung into the pleural space, increasing pressure within the space with every breath the patient takes.

THOMAS SPLINT: type of traction splint.

TRACTION: action of drawing or pulling on an object.

TRANSECTED: to cut transversely.

VASOMOTOR: affecting the size of a blood vessel.

VENOUS PRESSURE: pressure of the blood in the veins.

WHEEZING: whistling sounds made in breathing; a sign of spasm or narrowing of the bronchi.

INDEX

A

Abdomen:
  anatomy, 114–15
    of intrathoracic abdomen,
      115
    of retroperitoneal abdomen,
      115, 116
    of true abdomen, 115, 116
Abdominal trauma:
  in children, 168
  points to remember, 118–19
  types of injuries, 117
    blunt abdominal trauma, 117
    penetrating injuries, 117
  victim evaluation, 117–18
    examination, 118
    observation and history,
      117–18
  victim stabilization, 118

Abruptio placentae, 153
Acid burns, 143
  management of, 149
Actions at hospital, as stage of
    ambulance call, 24–25
Actions at scene, as stage of
    ambulance call, 24
Acute epidural hematoma, 105–6
Acute subdural hematoma, 106
Afterbirth. *See* Placenta.
Air bags:
  effect in frontal deceleration
    collisions, 10–11
  effect in lateral impact
    collisions, 12
Air splints, 129
Airway management:
  airway conscious patient, 56
  manual techniques for opening
    airway, 46–47

Airway management (*cont.*)
  chin lift, 46
  jaw lift, 46
  modified jaw thrust, 46
  mechanical techniques for
      opening airway, 48–52
    nasopharyngeal airway, 48–52
    oral airway, 48
  suctioning, 52
  unconscious patient, 57
  ventilation, 52–56
    bag-valve masks, 53–54
    mouth-to-mask ventilation,
      53
    mouth-to-mouth ventilation,
      52
    oxygen-powered breathing
      devices, 54
    spontaneously breathing
      patient, 54
  See also Upper airway
      management
Airway obstruction, 61
Alkali burns, 143
  management of, 149
Ambulance call:
  stages of, 23–25
    actions at hospital, 24–25
    actions at scene, 24
    dispatch stage, 23
    predispatch stage, 23
    travel to hospital, 24
    travel to scene, 23
Amputations, 123–24
Anaphylactic shock, 76
Ankle fractures, 138
Anoxic brain injuries, 103
Antishock garment, 81–84
  cardiac tamponade and, 72
  contraindications for use, 81,
      206

flail chest and, 67
  indications for use, 81, 206
  MAST survey, 37, 231
  myocardial contusion and, 70
  with no pressure gauges, 82
  with one pressure gauge, 83
  points to remember, 82
  principle of use, 81–82
  procedures for use, 201–6
    application, 201–4
    application to victim
      requiring traction splint,
      205
    deflation of trousers, 205–6
    inflation of trousers, 204
    points to remember, 205–6
  with two pressure gauges, 83
Aortic disruption, 73
Assessment of trauma. *See*
      Trauma assessment
Assessment priorities, 27, 225
Athletic competition, spinal cord
      trauma and, 90
Automobile accidents
  large accidents, 7–15
    auto-pedestrian accidents, 14
    children in, 13–14
    frontal deceleration
      collisions, 7–11
    lateral impact collisions,
      11–12
    rear impact collisions, 12–13
    rollover accidents, 13
    tractor accidents, 14–15
  small accidents, 15–17
    motorcycles, 15–16
    three-wheeled motor vehicles
      (ATVs), 16–17
  spinal cord trauma and, 89
Auto-pedestrian accidents, motion
      injury in, 14

B

Bag-valve masks, 53–54, 164
    upper airway management and,
        178–80
Basic EMT (Emergency Medical
        Technician), function of,
        2–3
Basic Trauma Life Support
        Primary Survey, 35, 233
Basic Trauma Life Support
        Secondary Survey, 38–39,
        239–43
Blast injury. *See* Explosion injury
Bleeding, primary survey and,
        231
Blunt abdominal trauma, 117
    in pregnancy, 157
B-point restraint, 11
Brain injuries, 104–6
    cerebral contusion, 104
    concussion, 104
    intercranial hemorrhage, 105–6
    See also Intercranial
        hemorrhage
Burns:
    anatomy/physiology, 140
    assessment of, 146–49
        depth, 147
        extent, 147–48
        general rule, 149
        history, 146
        patients requiring
            hospitalization, 148
        patients requiring transport
            to burn unit, 148–49
    associated injuries, 144–46
        carbon monoxide poisoning,
            145–46
        explosion injury, 146
        smoke inhalation, 144–45

chemical burns, 143
    management of, 149–51
in children, 168
electrical burns, 143–44
    management of, 151–52
management of, 149–51
pathophysiology, 141–42
    first-degree burns, 141
    second-degree burns, 141
    third-degree burns, 141–42
rule of nines, 147
thermal burns, 142–43
    management of, 149
types of, 142–44
upper airway injury, 142, 144
See also specific types of burns

C

Capillary blanch test, 78
Car accidents. *See* Automobile
        accidents
Carbon monoxide poisoning, 54,
        145–46
Cardiac tamponade, 70–72
    diagnosis, 72
        physical findings, 172
    pathophysiology, 70–72
    treatment, 72
Cardiogenic shock, 75
Catecholamines, 76–88, 92
Central cord syndrome, 93, 94
Cerebral contusion, 104
Cervical spine, 15, 86
Cervical strain. *See* Whiplash
Chemical burns, 15, 143
    in children, 164
    management of, 149–51
Chest, anatomy of, 59–61
Chest trauma, 54, 59–74
    airway obstruction, 61

Chest trauma (*cont.*)
  aortic disruption, 73
  cardiac tamponade, 70–72
  in children, 165
  diaphragmatic hernias, 73
  flail chest, 66–68
  impaled objects, 72
  massive hemothorax, 68–69
  myocardial contusion, 70
  open pneumothorax (sucking
    chest wound), 61–63
  pathophysiology, 61–73
  points to remember, 73–74
  simple pneumothorax, 73
  simple rib fractures, 73
  sternum fractures, 73
  tension pneumothorax, 64–66
  See also specific injuries
Child restraint seats, 13–14
Chin lift, 46, 47, 174, 175
Clark Pediatric Unit, 167
Clasp-knife effect, 10
Clavicle fractures, 10, 135, 136
Closed fractures, 120, 121
Coccyx, 86
Cold skin, as symptom of
    hypovolemic shock, 77
Collins hitch, 132, 196
Concussion, 104
Confusion:
  as symptom of hypovolemic
    shock, 77
  as symptom of spinal shock,
    79
Convulsions, head trauma and,
    111
Critical trauma situations, 169–72
  primary survey, 169–71
  secondary survey, 171–72
Cross chest-lap seat belt, 10
Cushing response, 102

D

Deep partial-thickness burns, 141
Dermis, definition of, 140
Diagnosis:
  cardiac tamponade, 72
    physical findings, 72
  flail chest, 67
    physical findings, 67
  massive hemothorax, 69
    physical findings, 69
  myocardial contusion, 70
  open pneumothorax, 62
  tension pneumothorax, 65
    physical findings, 65
Diaphragmatic hernias, 73
Dislocations, extremities, 123
Dispatch stage, of ambulance call,
    23
Diving accident:
  extraction of victim, 94
  spinal cord trauma and, 90
Donway traction splints, 199–200
Dorsal pedis pulse, 125
Driver, motion injury in frontal
    deceleration collisions, 7–8

E

Early hypovolemic shock, 77
  capillary blanch test, 78
Edema, as cause of upper airway
    obstruction, 45
Elbow fractures/dislocations, 135,
    137
Electrical burns, 143–44
  management of, 151–52
Electrical shock, spinal cord
    trauma and, 91
Emergency rapid extrication,
    189–93

objective, 189–93
  procedure, 190–93
  situations requiring, 189–90
Epidermis, definition of, 140
Explosion injury, 20, 146
Extremity trauma:
  assessment, 125–26
    general assessment, 126
    history, 125–26
  in children, 166–67
  injuries, 120–25
    amputations, 123–24
    dislocations, 123
    fractures, 120–23
    impaled objects, 125
    neurovascular injuries,
      124–25
    sprains/strains, 125
    wounds, 124
  management of, 126–37
    clavicle fractures, 135
    elbow fractures, 135
    femur fractures, 131
    foot fractures, 137
    forearm/wrist fractures,
      135–37
    hand fractures, 137
    hip fractures/dislocations,
      132
    knee fractures/dislocations,
      134
    pelvic fractures, 131
    shoulder fractures, 135
    spine fractures, 130
    splinting, 126–30
    tibia/fibula fractures, 134

F

Falls:
  spinal cord trauma and, 90

  vertical falls, 17–18
Femur fractures, 121, 131
Fetus, 153, 154
Fibula fractures, 134
Firearm injuries:
  high-velocity projectiles, 18
  low-velocity projectiles, 18–19
  shotgun wounds, 19
First-degree burns, 141
Flail chest, 66–68
  diagnosis, 67
    physical findings, 67
  pathophysiology, 66–67
  treatment, 67–68
Foot fractures, 137
Forearm fractures, 135–37, 138
Foreign bodies, as cause of upper
    airway obstruction, 45
Fractures:
  extremities, 120–23
  See specific bone fractures
Frontal deceleration collisions:
  injuries, 7–11
    driver, 7–8
      front-seat passenger, 8
      rear-seat passengers, 8–9
      restrained occupants, 9–11
  motorcycles, 15–16
Full thickness burns, 141

G

Glasgow Coma Scale, in head
    trauma in children, 166
Golden hour, 22, 23

H

Half-ring traction splints. *See*
    Thomas traction splints
Hand fractures, 137

Hare traction splints, 195–97
Head, anatomy of, 99–100
Head trauma, 54, 99–113
    anoxic brain injuries, 103
    in children, 166
    intercranial pressure, 102–3
    management of, 110–12
        potential problems, 111–12
        of victim with decreased
            LOC, 112
    pathophysiology, 100–102
    types of injuries, 103–6
        brain injuries, 104–6
        scalp wounds, 103
        skull injuries, 103–4
    victim evaluation, 107–10
        primary survey, 108–9
        secondary survey, 109–10
Helmet removal, procedures,
    207–10
Hematoma:
    epidural, 105–6
    subdural, 106
Hemorrhagic shock:
    flail chest and, 67
    See also Hypovolemic shock
Hemothorax, compared to tension
    pneumothorax, 70
Herniated invertebral disc, 91
High-velocity projectile wounds,
    18
Hip dislocation, mechanism of
    posterior dislocation, 132,
    133
Hip fractures, 132
Hyperextension (hyperflexion)
    injury, 13, 92, 93
Hyperventilation, use in head
    trauma in children, 166

Hypotension:
    as symptom of hypovolemic
        shock, 77
    as symptom of spinal shock, 79
Hypothermia, 92
Hypovolemic shock, 76–78, 80
    classification, 77–78
    early shock, 77
    late shock, 78
    management of, 80–81
    pathophysiology, 76–77
    symptoms, 77
Hypoxia, 55

I

Immobilization:
    of head and neck, 223
    spinal immobilization, 181–88
        candidates for, 181–82
        rigid extrication collar, 182,
            183, 186
        use of short backboard,
            182–84, 185
        when to immobilize, 182
Impaled objects:
    chest trauma caused by, 72
    extremities, 125
Inadequate air exchange:
    pathophysiology, 78
Infant restraint seats, 14
Intercranial hemorrhage, 105–6
    acute epidural hematoma,
        105–6
    acute subdural hematoma, 106
    intracerebral hemorrhage, 106,
        107
Intercranial pressure, 102–3

Intestines, protrusion through
wounds, 117, 119
Intracerebral hemorrhage, 106,
107
Intrathoracic abdomen, 60, 115

J

Jaw lift, 46, 47, 174, 175
Jaw thrust, 175
Joint dislocations, 123

K

Kendrick Extrication Device,
(K.E.D.), 186
Klippel traction splints, 197
Knee fractures/dislocations, 134
Knife wounds, 20

L

Lateral impact collisions:
motion injury and, 11–12
motorcycles, 16
Level of consciousness, head
trauma and, 108–9
Long backboard, 191, 192–93
procedures for use, 211–23
immobilizing head and neck,
223
logrolling prone victim,
214–18
logrolling supine victim,
211–14
securing backboard to
standing victim, 220–23
securing victim to backboard,
218–20

Lower airways, anatomy of, 45
Lower leg fractures, 135
Low-velocity projectile wounds,
18–19
Lumbar spine, 17, 86

M

Massive hemothorax, 68–69
diagnosis, 69
physical findings, 69
pathophysiology, 68 69
treatment, 69
MAST survey, 37, 231
Military antishock trousers
(MAST). *See* Antishock
garment
Modified jaw thrust, 46, 173, 174
Motion injury:
blast injury, 20
cause of, 4
large motor vehicle accidents,
7–15
auto-pedestrian accidents, 14
children in, 13–14
frontal deceleration
collisions, 7–11
lateral impact collisions,
11–12
rear impact collisions, 12–13
rollover accidents, 13
tractor accidents, 14–15
laws of physics relating to, 4
mechanisms of, 4–21
projectile penetration, 18–20
firearms, 18–19
knives, 20
small motor vehicle accidents,
15–17

Motion injury (*cont.*)
    motorcycles, 15–16
     three-wheeled motor vehicles
      (ATVs), 16–17
    vertical falls, 17–18
Motorcycle accidents:
  frontal deceleration collisions,
    15–16
  lateral impact collisions, 16
  rear impact collisions, 16
  three-wheeled motorcycles
    (ATVs), 16–17
Motor examination, for spinal
    cord trauma, 94
Motor vehicle accidents. *See*
    Automobile accidents
Mouth-to-mask ventilation, 53
Mouth-to-mouth ventilation, 52
  in pediatric trauma, 164
Myocardial contusion, 70
  diagnosis, 70
  pathophysiology, 70, 71
  treatment, 70

N

Nasal cannulas, 55
Nasopharyngeal airway, 48–52,
    176
  insertion of, 50, 51
National Emergency Medical
    Services Systems Act, 2
Neurogenic shock. *See* Spinal
    shock
Neurovascular injuries,
    extremities, 124–25
Nonrebreathing mask, 55

O

Obstructed airway algorithm, 42,
    253

Open fractures, 120, 121
Open pneumothorax (sucking
    chest wound), 61–63
  diagnosis, 62
  pathophysiology, 61–62
  treatment, 62–63
Oral airway, insertion of, 49
Oropharyngeal airway, 48, 178,
    179
Oxygen administration, general
    rules for, 55–56
Oxygen-powered breathing
    devices, 54

P

Pallor, as symptom of
    hypovolemic shock, 77
Parrot phrases:
  for primary survey, 36–37,
    232–35
  for secondary survey, 39–40,
    244–45
PASG. *See* Antishock garment
Pathophysiology:
  burns, 141–42
   first-degree burns, 141
   second-degree burns, 141
   third-degree burns, 141–42
  cardiac tamponade, 70–72
  flail chest, 66–67
  head trauma, 100–102
  hypovolemic shock, 76–77
  inadequate air exchange, 78
  massive hemothorax, 68–69
  myocardial contusion, 70, 71
  open pneumothorax, 61–62
  spinal shock, 78–79
  tension pneumothorax, 64–65
Patient assessment, 26–27
  communications with medical
    control, 27

primary survey, 26
rapid patient assessment, 41
secondary survey, 26
transport decision and critical
    interventions, 26
Pediatric trauma:
    abdominal trauma, 168
    airway obstruction, 162–64
        chemical/thermal burns,
            164
        foreign body aspiration,
            163–64
        impact injuries to face/neck,
            164
    burns, 168
    chest trauma, 165
    Clark Pediatric Unit, 167
    considerations, 161–62
        airway and ventilation, 162
        blood pressure, 162
        heart rate, 162
        hypotensive values, 162
        respiratory rate, 161
    extremity trauma, 166–67
    general approach to, 168
    head trauma, 166
    mouth-to-mouth ventilation,
        164
    shock, 165
    spinal cord trauma, 165
Pedis pulse, 125
Pelvic fractures, 12, 121, 131
Pelvic structures, traction splints
    and, 194
Penetrating injuries:
    abdomen, 117
    in pregnancy, 157
    in spinal cord trauma, 91
Pericardial tamponade, 68, 73
Pericardium, 70
Pharyngeal airways:
    insertion of, 176–78

    nasopharyngeal airway, 176
    oropharyngeal airway, 178,
        179
Pillows, used as soft splints,
    130
Placenta, 153
    abruptio placentae, 153
Plastic face mask, 55
Pocket masks, 53
    upper airway management and,
        178, 180
Posterior dislocation of hip:
    mechanism of, 133
    splinting, 133
Predispatch stage, of ambulance
    call, 23
Pregnancy:
    anatomy/physiology, 153–54,
        155
        changes during pregnancy,
            154
Pregnancy trauma:
    blunt abdominal trauma, 157
    management of, 159–60
        oxygen administration, 159
        transport, 159–60
        volume replacement, 159
        vomiting, 159
    penetrating injuries, 157
    victim evaluation, 157–59
Primary survey, 224–35
    assessment priorities, 225
        evaluate airway, 225–26
        evaluate breathing and
            circulation, 226–29
        MAST survey, 231
        stop major bleeding, 231
    conducting of, 224
    critical injuries/conditions,
        231–32
    critical trauma situations,
        169–71

Primary survey (*cont.*)
head trauma, 108–9
level of consciousness, 108
vital signs, 108–9
procedure, 232–35
Basic Trauma Life Support
Primary Survey, 233
parrot phrases, 232–35
Projectile penetration, 18–20
firearms, 18–19
knives, 20

R

Radial pulse, 124
Rapid patient assessment:
ground rules for teaching and
testing, 246–47
obstructed airway algorithm,
253
patient assessment pearls,
247–48
procedure, 246
trauma scenario example,
249–50
grade sheet, 250–51
Rear impact collisions:
motion injury in, 12–13
motorcycles, 16
Rear-seat passenger, motion
injury in frontal
deceleration collisions, 8–9
Reflex examination, for spinal
cord trauma, 94
Respiration, mechanisms of, 92
Restrained occupants, motion
injury in frontal
deceleration collisions,
9–11
Retroperitoneal abdomen, 115,
116

Rib fractures, 73
Rigid extrication collar, 182, 183,
186, 191
Rigid splints, 128
Rollover accidents, motion injury
in, 13
Rule of nines, 147

S

Sacrum, 86
Sager traction splints, 198–99
Scene survey. *See* Primary survey;
Secondary survey
Seat belts/restraints, 10, 12, 13
Secondary survey, 236–45
conducting of, 236–38
contacting medical control,
238–39
critical trauma situations,
171–72
head trauma, 109–10
extremities, 109–10
pupils, 109
procedure, 239–45
Basic Life Support Secondary
Survey, 239–43
parrot phrases, 244–45
Second-degree burns, 141
Sensory examination, for spinal
cord trauma, 94
Septic shock, 76
Shock, 54, 75–84
anaphylactic shock, 76
antishock garment, 81–84
cardiogenic shock, 75
causes of, 75–76
failure of pump, 75
lack of adequate air
exchange, 76

lack of adequate vascular
  system, 76
lack of fluid volume, 75
in children, 165
definition of, 75
head trauma and, 112
hypovolemic shock, 76–78, 80
inadequate air exchange, 78
septic shock, 76
spinal shock, 78–79, 80
victim evaluation, 79–80
Short backboard, 182–84, 185
Shotgun wounds, 19
Shoulder fractures/dislocations,
  135, 136
Simple pneumothorax, 73
Simple rib fractures, 73
Skin, layers of, 140
Slings/swathes, used as soft
  splints, 130
Smoke inhalation, 54, 144–45
Soft splints, 128–30
  air splints, 129
  pillows, 130
  slings/swathes, 130
  vacuum splints, 129
Spanish windlass, 132, 196
Spinal column, anatomy of, 86
Spinal cord, 87–89
  relationship to vertebra, 89
Spinal cord trauma, 85–98
  brief neurological examination,
    93–94
  causes of, 89–91
    athletic competition, 90
    diving accident, 90
    electrical shock, 91
    fall, 90
    motor vehicle accident, 89
    penetrating trauma, 91

sudden twist, 91
in children, 165
fractures/dislocations, 87–88
management of, 96–98
mechanism of injury, 90
priority plan, 95–96
  arrival at scene, 95
  initial assessment, 95–96
specific injuries, 91–93
  central cord syndrome, 93, 94
  hypothermia, 92
  spinal shock, 92
  whiplash, 92, 93
Spinal immobilization, 181–88
  objectives, 181–84
    candidates for
      immobilization, 181–82
    use of short backboard,
      182–84, 185
    when to immobilize, 182
  points to remember, 184–86
  rigid extrication collar, 182,
    183, 186
Spinal shock, 92
  management of, 80–81
  pathophysiology, 78–79
  symptoms, 79
Spine fractures, 130
Splints:
  general rules, 127–28
  lower leg fractures, 135
  purpose of, 126
  reasons for use, 126
  types of, 128–30
    rigid splints, 128
    soft splints, 128–30
    traction splints, 130
  when to use, 126–27
Spontaneously breathing patients:
  ventilation for, 54, 55

Spontaneously breathing patients (*cont.*)
    nasal cannulas, 55
    nonrebreathing mask, 55
    plastic face mask, 55
Sprains/strains, extremities, 125
Sternum fractures, 73
Sucking chest wound. *See* Open pneumothorax
Suctioning, airway management, 52
Superficial partial-thickness burns, 141
Sweating, as symptom of hypovolemic shock, 77
Swelling. *See* Edema

T

Tachycardia, as symptom of hypovolemic shock, 77
Tachypnea, as symptom of spinal shock, 79
Tension pneumothorax, 64–66
  compared to hemothorax, 70
  diagnosis, 65
    physical findings, 65
  pathophysiology, 64–65
  treatment, 65–66
Thermal burns, 142–43
  in children, 164
  management of, 149
Third-degree burns, 141–42
Thirst, as symptom of hypovolemic shock, 77
Thomas traction splints, 195
Thoracic spine, 86, 89
Thorax, 60–61
Three-point seat restraint, 10
Three-wheeled motorcycles (ATVs), motion injuries and, 16–17

Tibia fractures, 134
Tibial pulse, 125
Tongue, as cause of upper airway obstruction, 43–45
Tourniquet, 124
Traction splints, 130
  application of, 130
  application of antishock garment to victim requiring, 205
  Donway splints, 199–200
  hare splints, 195–97
  Klippel splints, 197
  purpose of, 194
  Sager splints, 198–99
  Thomas splints, 195
Tractor accidents, motion injury in, 14–15
Trauma:
  assessment, 25–31
    patient assessment and management, 26–27
    preliminary actions at scene, 25
    priorities, 27
    priority plan, 27–31
  questions to ask at scene, 5
  statistics, 1
  victim evaluation, 22–42
Trauma assessment:
  assessment priorities, 27, 225
  Basic Trauma Life Support Primary Survey, 35
  Basic Trauma Life Support Secondary Survey, 38–39
  contacting medical control, 34
  critical injuries/conditions, 31–32
  MAST survey, 37
  Obstructed Airway Algorithm, 42

parrot phrases for primary
    survey, 36–37
parrot phrases for secondary
    survey, 39–40
patient assessment, 26–27
    communications with medical
        control, 27
    primary survey, 26
    secondary survey, 26
    transport decision and critical
        interventions, 26
patient management, steps in,
        26
preliminary actions at scene, 25
    equipment, 25
    scene survey, 25
priority plan, 27–32
rapid patient assessment, 41
secondary survey, 32–34
Travel to hospital, as stage of
    ambulance call, 24
Travel to scene, as stage of
    ambulance call, 23
Treatment:
    cardiac tamponade, 72
    flail chest, 67–68
    massive hemothorax, 69
    myocardial contusion, 70
    open pneumothorax, 62–63
    tension pneumothorax, 65–66
True abdomen, 115, 116
T-strap, 132, 196

                    U

Upper airway, anatomy of, 43, 44
Upper airway management, 142,
        144, 173–80
    bag-valve mask, 178–80
    insertion of pharyngeal airways,
        176–78

    nasopharyngeal airway, 176
    oropharyngeal airway, 178,
        179
    manual techniques to open
        airway, 173–74
        chin lift, 174, 175
        jaw lift, 174, 175
        jaw thrust, 175
        modified jaw thrust, 173, 174
    objectives, 173
    obstructions, 43–44
        edema (swelling), 45
        foreign bodies, 45
        tongue, 43–45
    pocket mask with supplemental
        oxygen, 178, 180
    procedures, 173–80
    suctioning of airway, 174–76
Uterus, 153, 154
    See also Pregnancy trauma

                    V

Vacuum splints, 129
Ventilation:
    for spontaneously breathing
        patients, 54, 55
    See also Airway management;
        Upper airway management
Verbal responses, Glasgow coma
        scale, 162
Vertebral foramen, 87, 89
Vertical falls, motion injury in,
        17–18
Victim evaluation:
    abdominal trauma, 117–18
        examination, 118
        observation and history,
            117–18
    head trauma, 107–10
        primary survey, 108–9

Victim evaluation (*cont.*)
    secondary survey, 109–10
  in pregnancy trauma, 157–59
  trauma, 22–42
Vital signs, head trauma and,
    108–9
Volume replacement, for pregnant
    trauma victim, 159
Vomiting:
  head trauma and, 111–12
  pregnancy trauma and, 159

W

Weakness:
  as symptom of hypovolemic
    shock, 77
  as symptom of spinal shock,
    79
Whiplash, 13, 92, 93
Womb. *See* Uterus
Wounds, extremities, 124
Wrist fractures, 138